Healthy by *Design*

Pray Powerfully, Lose Weight

(Reflections of God's Love)

21-Days of short prayers, declarations, scriptures and quotes for a healthy body, spirit, and soul.

Cathy Morenzie

Guiding Light Publishing

First Edition (as Reflections of God's Love): September 2016

Second Edition (as Pray Powerfully, Lose Weight): December 2019

ISBN: 978-1-9992207-1-6 Print

978-1-9992207-2-3 Digital

Publishing by Guiding Light Publishing
261 Oakwood Ave, York, ON, Canada, M6E 2V3

Note: The information in this book is for educational purposes only and is not recommended as a means of diagnosing or treating illness. All situations concerning physical or mental health should be supervised by a health professional knowledgeable in treating that particular condition. Neither the author nor anyone affiliated with Healthy by Design dispenses medical advice nor do they prescribe any remedies or assume any responsibility for anyone who chooses to treat themselves.

Cover Design by: kimmontefortedesign.com

Cover and author photo by: Martin Brown Photography

Interior Design by: Davor Dramikanin

This book is dedicated with deepest love and respect
to all the courageous women who have participated in the
'Weight Loss, God's Way Challenge'.
You have been as much as a blessing
and inspiration, as I trust, the challenge has been for you.

Table of Contents

A Note From the Author

You're about to change your life! As you embark on this weight loss and faith journey, I couldn't be more excited for you and honored to provide you with this indispensable tool to support you on your journey.

Every day, people like you change how they have been approaching their weight loss programs. They share how our *Healthy by Design* books and *Weight Loss, God's Way* online programs have transformed their lives, from reaching their weight goals to increasing their sense of worthiness and self-confidence, while also deepening their relationship with their Heavenly Father.

This book promises to deliver the same results. It will lay the foundation for weight loss, God's way— prayer!. Prayer truly is the answer and that's what you'll discover.

To give you a head start, I'm also offering you these special gifts to you just for purchasing this book:

Enjoy our **Top 10 Prayers** for your health and weight loss. They are designed to help you focus your prayers and point you towards Christ, where you can align with Him and His best for you. You can print them out and post to remind you of God's promises, save them as a screen saver on your phone or computer, or share them with your friends on social media.

3 Steps to Overcome Emotional Eating – How to overcome emotional eating with God's help. Use this repeatable 3-step approach to reverse impulsive eating habits and turn your needs over to God instead. Join my free newsletter to receive this lesson directly in your inbox and join the 10,000+ Christian women releasing their weight for good, God's Way.

www.praypowerfullyloseweightbonus.com

Praying for your success,

Cathy Morenzie

www.cathymorenzie.com

PRINCIPLES FOR PERMANENT WEIGHT LOSS

"I'm finally getting it. After all these years of 'trying' to lose weight, I finally see that it's not really about the weight at all. Now it makes sense why the more I tried, the more I failed."

"I need to unlearn everything I know about weight loss and retrain myself to do less and trust God more. He made us, after all, so it makes perfect sense to seek Him for instructions of how to live a healthy life."

"I can see I am taking steps to change and to put God at the center of my journey to building Him a temple worthy of His greatness. I stand in His Grace as I move in baby steps and am beginning to truly understand that He does not make mistakes and my size (about 60 lbs.) is not a mistake but rather a reflection of me standing in my own strength for too long."

"As I saw myself in a glass mirror today at work, I said to myself, I love me; I'm changing; I have a new attitude; I am training hard, 5-6 days/wk, and making better lifestyle health/eating choices. And, I'm loving the process! I'm loving my life. I can finally say that after so many years— not because I've reached my goals...but because I'm in the process, the trenches of achieving my goals. And that's what I love!!! Ha! I'm finally in that zone. God does answer prayers!"

"Just finished the 21-Day Challenge and was so blessed by it! It really pushed me to look inside myself for the things holding me back and to then seek the Lord in receiving that breakthrough!"

~ Weight Loss, God's Way Challenge participants

So what has made the difference for these women and the tens of thousands more like them who are finally feeling empowered and free? It was not finding the right diet or the right exercise program. It was not learning how to count calories or how to resist temptation. What made the difference for them was learning to LET GO.

Learning to LET GO of all of their preconceived notions about how they should lose weight.

Learning to LET GO of their need to control everything and everyone, which kept them overwhelmed and overweight.

Learning to LET GO of their perfectionism that would never allow them to make a mistake or slip up.

Learning to LET GO of their fears, their limiting beliefs, and their blaming, excuse-making, procrastinating, and negative thoughts.

Learning to LET GO of their need to stuff and pacify their feelings with food and instead allow themselves to feel what they've been avoiding.

They discovered how to let it all go and entrust it all to God. They were finally able to cease striving (Psalms 46:10), cast their cares on God (1 Peter 5:7) and let Him fight their battles (Exodus 14:14).

And that same peace, freedom and empowerment is available to you, too, through this devotional guide. It will guide you to the only true way to release weight and keep it off without guilt, shame and judgement. It will teach you the power of prayer and its power to transform you from the inside out. It will guide you to God's truth about your health and your weight so you can LET GO and let God do the healing work that He wants to do in your life.

What is 'Pray Powerfully, Lose Weight'?

This book is created for you if you:

- **Want to strengthen your prayer life**

- Want to **lose weight, God's way**

- **Are tired of dieting** and want to lose weight in a way that aligns with your values as a Christian woman (or man)

- Want to gain a **deeper understanding of** why you've been spinning your wheels

- Are not sure **how to pray** for your **health** and **weight loss**

- Want to **discover all the factors holding you back** from achieving your healthy weight and learn how to truly submit them to God.

- Want to develop a **consistent** and **effective** routine of **praying for your health**

Pray Powerfully, Lose Weight is a beautiful collection of short weight-loss-related devotionals, prayers, declarations, scriptures, and quotes designed to teach you how to pray for your weight loss.

By the end of this book, you will feel confident in the power of your prayers. You will feel your faith rise and your fears decrease. You will begin to feel hopeful again. You will gain the confidence to 'ask whatever in His name, and He will do it' (John 14:13).

How is this weight loss devotional different?

If I told you that everything you were doing to try to lose weight was wrong, would you change?

If I told you that the more you try to lose weight the more you will probably end up gaining, would you stop dieting?

If I told you that weight loss is an emotional issue that must be dealt with on a spiritual level and not on a nutritional (eat less) or physical (exercise more) level, would you believe me?

Most of us would probably try to change for a little while, but eventually we would end up in the same place. Why? There are five main reasons.

1. We are not prepared for the amount of work it will take to truly change.

2. Deep down we don't really believe that we can change.

3. We are limited by our life's experiences, which are not indicative of achieving success (at least in the area of weight loss).

4. We do not have a system to get us from point 'a' to point 'b'.

5. We are gripped by our fears and they stop us dead in our tracks.

This devotional is different because it not just a bunch of scriptures put together about the benefits of prayer. It's the result of years of seeing the power of prayer first-hand in the lives of tens of thousands of women as a result of the principles in this book.

When you read these devotions you, too, will:

- Discover how the power of prayer can transform your weight loss

- Understand the importance of praying for your weight loss

- Learn to develop a consistent routine of praying for your weight loss

- Get clarity and focus from spending time each day with the Lord

- Study what the Bible says about weight loss

- Learn how to prioritize your weight loss based on God's Word

"It's really not about your weight at all."

When it comes to our weight, more than achieving a number on the scale, we want to be FREE. Free from obsessing about our weight; free from having to measure food, plan food, make time to go to the gym, weigh in, eat emotionally, stress over what we're going to wear and what we're going to cook for dinner.

We want to be led by the Holy Spirit so that we are so in tune with His leading that our health is no longer even on our radar. It happens as a natural outpouring of loving our Heavenly Father. It happens when we spend time with Him and learn to seek His best for us in prayer and communion with Him.

We want to eat when we're hungry and stop when we're full. We want to eat right and exercise as a natural expression of showing glory to our Father. We want to eat to fuel our bodies and not for temporary emotional soothing. We want to be motivated to be healthy instead of feeling burdened by our 'should list'— 'I should exercise', 'I should eat healthy', and 'I should pray more'. Contrary to what you may have been taught, this freedom does not come through traditional weight loss programs. If you've dieted then you know that they make you feel bound, trapped, guilty, condemned and hopeless.

The freedom we're searching for is understanding and accepting God's overwhelming and steadfast love for us as we spend time with Him. As we learn to give and receive it, all the other cares of this world will fall away. When prayer is the foundation of all we do, the Holy Spirit will strip everything else away—even the excess weight. What will be left is a life of gratitude, peace, joy, and love rooted in a wonderful relationship with our Heavenly Father.

"Let all that you do be done in love."
(1 Corinthians 14:16)

Take time each day as you read this devotional to search out the true condition of your heart. Commit to letting go all of your faulty beliefs about what you think it takes to lose weight and submit them to God in prayer. Ask the Holy Spirit to illuminate any parts of your life that are 'should-driven' rather than 'spirit-driven'. Draw closer to God each day and cast your cares on Him (1 Peter 5:7). Remember, it's in fellowshipping with Him each day and allowing His spirit to lead you that your health will be restored with the fullness of God's love for you.

The Healthy by Design Principles

God has given us immutable laws and principles to govern our lives. These principles apply to every person, every situation, and every circumstance. Even if you do not practice them per se, you will still experience the consequences if you go against them. These five principles are reinforced in all of the *Healthy by Design* books (and weightlossgodsway.com programs). Use these principles in your weight releasing journey and other areas of your life to experience the victory, freedom, and peace that God has already given you.

1. Identification: Good health is your identity, not your destination (Gen. 1:27).

You were created to be in good health—after all, you were created in God's image. Think about that for a minute ... you were created in God's image!

The Bible says, *"Then God said, 'Let Us make man in Our image, according to Our likeness; and let them rule over the fish of the sea and over the birds of the sky and over the cattle and over all the earth, and over every creeping thing that creeps on the earth.' God created man in His own image, in the image of God He created him; male and female He created them* (Genesis 1:26-27 NASB).

So if that's true, then why have you spent so many years of your adult life trying to get to a specific number on the scale? Just think about the wasted energy, time, frustration, and happiness you've lost trying to achieve something you already possess.

Soooooo the message here is to: Stop trying so hard to work at something you already possess. Focus on trusting God more and trying less. Stop being afraid of success. Success is in your DNA—it's who you are!

Stop chasing a mythical, magical illusion of what you think your life would look like at a certain weight. It's time to see and accept the awesomeness of who you are right now. Without acceptance it will be difficult, if not impossible, to make progress.

Stop waiting, wishing, wanting, hoping, praying, and wasting time worrying about the future. God is a right now God; He is here in the present, guiding you step by step. I know, easier said than done. But as you begin to trust that good health is part of your identity, then you will stop wasting so much time searching for a magical, mythical fantasy that doesn't exist and begin to embrace who God has called you to be—regardless of your current size.

2. Ternion (triad): Good health involves a combination of healing your body, soul, and spirit (1 Thess. 5:23).

God made us distinct and unique from all of creation. Because we were created in God's image, He also created us with a tripartite nature like himself. As God encompasses the Father,

Son, and Holy Spirit, we too are composed of three parts. Our spirit, soul, and body.

As human beings we live in a physical body, we have a soul, and we live eternally as a spirit that connects with God's Spirit.

Our tripartite nature works to keep us healthy and whole. It's impossible to address one area without giving attention to the other.

The Bible says, *"Now may the God of peace Himself sanctify you entirely; and may your spirit and soul and body be preserved complete, without blame at the coming of our Lord Jesus Christ"* (1 Thessalonians 5:23 NASB).

For us to be in total health as God intended, all three parts of our being need to be healthy. They are intertwined and interconnected. Here's how:

Body

Our body is our outer shell, but it houses the temple of the living God. It is your physical being. It consists of our five senses: taste, touch, sight, smell, and hearing. In His infinite wisdom, God created our bodies to operate in harmony with our souls and spirits. If our physical bodies are not healthy, it negatively impacts our spirits and our souls.

Here's what the Bible teaches us about our physical bodies:

It houses the living God (1Cor 3:16-17).

We are to present it to God as a living sacrifice (Romans 12:2).

We are to put no confidence in it (Phil 3:3).

We are to discipline it and keep it under control (1 Cor 9:27).

Soul

Our souls are made up of our conscious and subconscious minds, which house our thoughts, conscience, will, and emotions. It gives us our personality. This is where the battle rages. It's where we experience the anxiety, doubts, and fears which manifest in our bodies as excess weight and illness. If our soul is bound then we will have difficulty honoring our temples, and we will have difficulty connecting with God.

Here's what the Bible teaches us about our souls:

The Lord created us a living soul (Gen 2:7).

It is immortal (Matt 10:28).

It is in conflict with our spirit (1 Cor 2:14).

They can lead us away and lead to sin and death (James 1:13-15).

Spirit

At our core is our spirit; it's the part of us that connects with God. This is our contact point with God, where our spirit communicates with His. Paul says, *"When we cry 'Abba! Father' it's the Spirit Himself bearing witness with our spirit that we are children of God."* (Romans 8:15-17.) It's only when we align our spirits with our Heavenly Father's that we will ever be successful at anything we do, including getting healthier.

Here's what the Bible teaches us about our spirits:

God enlightens our spirit so we can know truth (Proverbs 20:27).

The indwelling Spirit of Christ dwells in our heart (Romans 8:16).

God's word can divide our soul and spirit (Heb 4:12).

Key takeaway: We are tripartite beings. Whatever happens to one part of our being has repercussions in the other two areas.

3. Revelation: Information without revelation is meaningless (Rom 8:5, Rom 12:2, James 1:5).

Here's an obvious, but important, question. Do you need more information on weight loss? Didn't think so. You probably already have more information than you can ever read. The problem is not a lack of information, but the exact opposite.

Most of us suffer from information overload. You probably have books sitting on your bookshelf or table that you mean to read, emails that you need to respond to, and interesting articles that you one day hope to skim.

Most women I talk to are so overwhelmed that I know for sure that the answer you're looking for isn't found in reading another book or signing up for another program.

Information in and of itself is meaningless. Ask yourself the following questions about all the information you've gathered to date.

Revelation comes from the Holy Spirit. It doesn't come from our wisdom or intellect. In fact, it's our intellect that keeps getting us into trouble. We 'think' we know more than God, so we keep taking matters back into our own hands. James 1:5 reminds us that it is God who gives us wisdom.

1. Are you applying it?

What good is it to say you trust God with your health, yet never submit the journey to Him or never run to Him in your time of need? It's one thing to read something in the Bible or even in a book, but without relying on the power of the Holy Spirit to transform us it's just information, which has no power on its own. Remember this: Knowledge is NOT power. Application of knowledge is power.

2. Have you mastered it?

I remember signing up for one of those online 30-day squat challenges. I got up to day four and quit. Yet if someone asked me, I would probably say, "Yeah, I've done it before." That's what many of us do. We invest in something and quit before we've achieved results, yet we talk like we're now experts on the subject.

I have a similar challenge with tracking my food. Yes, I track it, but am I using the tool effectively to eat within my daily allowance or as an effective tool for weight-management?

The answer is no, so until then I will continue using it until I learn what I need to learn from the tool. Don't get frustrated or give up if you miss a few days or if you can't stick to it. Keep on trying until you master it.

3. Do your results prove it?

This is the biggest test of true knowledge. I remember strik-ing up a conversation with this marketing 'guru' who began telling me about a new miracle fat-loss pill that has been sell-ing like hotcakes. He told me all the benefits of the product and how amazing it was, and was about 50 pounds overweight! Or have you ever had the sister at church tell you a Word of the Lord for you, yet her life was in shambles?

Let your results speak louder than your words. Results never lie. If you're not getting results in your weight-loss program, stop wasting time gathering more useless information.

4. Transformation: Transformation comes through daily submission (2 Cor 10:5, Luke 9:23).

Let's face it, sacrificing anything isn't pleasant at the time. Even the word itself conjures up feelings of pain and struggle. Yet our Bible teaches us that living a life of sacrifice is the only way to enjoy a life of freedom in Christ. In Matthew 10:39, Jesus says, *"Whoever finds his life will lose it, and whoever loses his life for my sake will find it."*

The reality is that many of us are frustrated and feel utter-ly hopeless with our current state of health, but are unwilling to make the necessary sacrifices it takes to achieve a healthy weight. We've been struggling with our weight for most of our lives and it feels like things will never change. Despite our feel-ings of hopelessness, we keep grasping at short-term worldly solutions to end our pain. We keep trying solution after solu-tion, but they eventually get too difficult, time-consuming, or we just get bored and move on to the next thing.

It's only when we can embrace Jesus' teaching that short-term sacrifice will lead to long-term fulfillment, and the concept of sacrificial living will not be so daunting.

The solution is found in God. Until we know the true heart of God, sacrifice will always seem like deprivation or punishment, but it's the exact opposite. Freedom is found in dying to ourselves every hour of every day so that we can live an abundant life.

1. God calls us to submission because He understands how easily we are led away by our flesh if we don't exercise restraint.

He knows our propensity to make idols out of everything, and how these idols will turn our attention away from Him.

> *"No one can serve two masters. Either you will hate the one and love the other, or you will be devoted to the one and despise the other. You cannot serve both God and money."*
> (Matthew 6:24)

2. God calls us to submission because He knows that our insatiable desires for food (money, power, sex) will always keep us wanting even more. We try to fill our needs with worldly things instead of Godly things, so no matter how much food we eat we will always want more. No matter how much money we make we will always want more (or whatever your weakness is).

> *"But each one is tempted when he is carried away and enticed by his own lust. Then when lust has conceived, it gives birth to sin; and when sin is accomplished, it brings forth death..."*
> (James 1:14-15)

3. God calls us to submission because He knows that He is the only one who can fulfill all of our needs. When we sacrifice our appetites and draw closer to God He honors our actions, meets us in our time of need, and draws closer to us. Satiety and satisfaction are found in Him alone.

> *"Blessed are those who hunger and thirst for*
> *righteousness, for they will be filled."*
> (Matthew 5:6)

As you read this book you begin to embrace your weight loss journey as a marathon, not a sprint. You will realize the futility of searching for the quick fixes and easy answers and finally grasp that there is no such thing.

You simply can't cram what the Holy Spirit is trying to teach you on this journey. It's not like a high school test. You're on the journey of your life, and it will take time and patience.

Change is a daily process. It's the little things that you do daily that will get you to your goals.

Every time you say 'yes' to God, you will move closer to your goal.

5. Action: You must move past the natural resistance from contemplation to action (Jas 1:22; Jas 2:26).

What do I mean by natural resistance?

Resistance refers to the trials, roadblocks, difficulties, frustrations, set-backs, and hindrances you encounter on your journey. It could be anything from backsliding, self-sabotage, an injury, an illness in the family, traveling, vacation, family visiting, unexpected company, or anything that slows down or stops your weight loss. Some of this resistance is God perfecting us, some is the enemy trying to keep us from fulfilling God's promises for us, and some is the result of our faulty thinking and poor choices. Wherever the resistance comes from, we all must move through it.

When we experience resistance, most of us usually do one of two things: We either dig our heels in deeper or we quit. What if I told you that neither of these options is correct? Resistance is not to be fought. Think of quicksand—the more you resist, the faster you sink. The resistance is to be released to God so that we can 'cast our cares on Him' as we find the courage to take action.

Instead of always 'getting ready to get ready', planning to start your new diet on 'Monday', or doing more research on the right program for you, stop procrastinating and take action already. That's what this last principle means and that's what you'll begin to discover how to do.

How to use this book

I suggest you read through the 21 days, one day at a time. This is not the type of book to read in one sitting. You will miss the gold that God has for you in the pages of this book.

Each of the 21 days contains eight sections: devotion, action, validation, meditation, inspiration, declaration, supplication, and reflection. Below are some instructions on how to use each of these sections. Don't feel like you need to do all of them each day.

Devotion:

*"So we have come to know and to believe the love
that God has for us. God is love, and whoever abides
in love abides in God, and God abides in him."*
(1 John 4:16)

The devotion introduces the main topic in both a practical and spiritual context. Read it to understand how God wants you to pray yourself through every aspect of your life, which includes your weight loss. Each devotion is designed to bring you back to the overarching truth, that God loves you and wants you to spend time with you in prayer, so you can get filled with His love! It's in fellowship with Him that we experience the power of His love that will heal and transform us. It's when we step out of God's love that we struggle with our health and our weight. Let God's love fill you as you read the devotional every day. Once you've completed the devotion, write out a prayer to God to help you in this area.

Action:

In this section you will be guided to take action by praying for a specific area of your weight loss journey. Take some time and journal your prayers to God, sharing your heart with Him.

If you are need additional guidance or inspiration on how to pray for the specific area of your weight loss journey, you can refer to the prayers at the back of the book in the appendix.

Validation:

*"Therefore encourage one another and build one
another up, just as you are doing."*
(1 Thessalonians 5:11)

Knowing that we are not alone on this journey gives us a sense of comfort. Knowing that our experiences are not unique to us alone gives a sense of hope that, if others have shared our struggles and made it through, we can, too. There is power in numbers.

Read the comments and testimonies shared by other women to inspire you and let you know that your feelings and experiences are valid and not unique to you. You are not alone.

Meditation:

*"Oh, how I love your law!
I meditate on it all day long."*
(Psalm 119:97)

Take the daily scripture with you as you go about your day. Write it down, ask the Holy Spirit to bring it to your remembrance when appropriate. Put it on your fridge or on the dashboard of your car—anywhere you will be able to refer to it a few times a day. At the end of this book you will find all of the scriptures for you to print or cut out and take with you each day.

Inspiration:

*"An intelligent heart acquires knowledge, and the
ear of the wise seeks knowledge."*
(Proverbs 18:15)

Sometimes, taking God's Word out of a spiritual context and putting it into another context gives it a whole new meaning. It also reminds us that God's Word is universal, and spans every facet of life. Learn what some of the world's great thought leaders have to say about these topics.

Declaration:

*"Keep listening to my words, and let my
declaration be in your ears."*
(Job 13:17)

The Word of God has the power to transform our lives. I suggest you open your mouth and speak this declaration out loud. Listen to yourself as you speak. Pray for the faith to believe what you're saying. At the end of this book you will find all of the declarations. Print or cut them out, and post them in various places in your home, car, or place of work.

Supplication:

*"Do not be anxious about anything, but in every
situation, by prayer and petition, with thanksgiving,
present your requests to God."*
(Philippians 4:6)

The foundation of this book can be found here—prayer! To supplicate means to ask humbly and earnestly, or simply put to prayer. Many of us have never thought of asking God to help us on this journey. We feel we are not entitled because we do not have the right, or because we feel we are being disobedient to Him. We often go to Him, begging or feeling ashamed or un-worthy, or perhaps we simply never thought of praying for our weight loss.

Use these prayers as a powerful tool to allow you to go be-fore God, and pray in agreement with His Word and His will for your life.

Reflection:

Life can get so busy. Even our devotion time can become something else to do on our to-do list. Taking time to reflect allows us to slow down and take some time to think about how the daily topics affect you and your relationship with God. The daily reflection will give you a better understanding of yourself in light of the Word of God. This will be a good section to read at the end of the day, after you have reflected on the scripture and carried out the daily action step.

Ready? Let's go!

Devotions

Day 1: Wed

PRAYER FOR THE JOURNEY

Devotion:

You're going to kick off this prayer challenge praying for the ability to set goals in line with God's best for you.

You've set so many goals for so many different things—especially your health over the years. That's why the thought of setting another one brings memories of failure and self-sabotage. So what will be different this time?

Answer: a commitment to pray yourself through your journey. You will develop a prayer life that includes communing with God BEFORE you begin your journey, DURING the challenging times of your journey, and AFTER you achieve your goal. You will continue to pray so you can maintain your progress.

Every time you take another step in prayer, with the Lord as your strength, you are changing from the inside-out, although it may not feel like it.

Through prayer in agreement with God, you will set goals in partnership with your heavenly Father—not based on society's unrealistic expectations, but based on your desire for seeking God's best for you.

In prayer, when you set your intention on getting healthier for God, you can't fail because you're trusting in God's strength, not your own limited abilities.

In prayer, you will line up your desires with God's (Proverbs 3:5-6). As you commit this process to prayer, your perspective will change from setting goals that are focused on you to setting goals based on what God can do through you. His love for you will help you set goals that will transform your life and your weight loss.

Action:

Pray for the ability to set goals in line with God's best for you.

Validation:

"I commit to pursuing Godly goals. I ask the Holy Spirit to help me live in line with His perfect goals for my weight loss and my life. It is my desire to bring You glory, as I lose weight and become healthier. Please help me as I begin this journey, dear Lord! Thank You!"

"I must keep this body healthy and strong. God is calling me to serve in ministry and I need to be healthy and strong. I want to serve my Lord Jesus wholeheartedly and I must get healthy."

"Wonderful beginning! I feel I was able to write realistic goals for my weight release that will be for my good and His glory!

Meditation:

*"Commit your actions to the LORD, and your
plans will succeed."*
(Proverbs 16:3 NLT)

Inspiration:

*Setting goals is the first step to turning the
invisible into the visible.*
~ Tony Robbins

Declaration:

I walk in wisdom to set realistic goals that glorify You. I submit my goals and plans to You and I trust You to show me the way. My goals align with my Heavenly Father's and are bathed in the Word of God. I declare that my goals will come to fruition. As I draw close to You, I am successful and victorious in the Name of Jesus.

Supplication:

Dear Lord, I want to glorify You in my body because it is Your temple. I submit myself and my goals to You. I know when I am in alignment with Your will and purpose for my life, I will be successful! Lord, give me the courage to take steps every day towards fulfilling my health goals and becoming the person You created me to be. In Your glorious name, I pray. Amen!

Reflection:

1. In what ways do you continually sabotage yourself when you set your goals? Take time to confess any goals that are not in line with the heart of God, as stated in Scripture.

> *"For I know the plans I have for you," declares the*
> *LORD, "plans to prosper you and not to harm you,*
> *plans to give you hope and a future."*
> (Jeremiah 29:11)

----

2. Invite God into your goal-setting this time. Ask Him to show you how He will be glorified when you are healthier. How much does He want you to weigh? How does He want you to go about reaching your goal?

_____

_____

_____

_____

_____

_____

3. Now commit yourself to pursuing Godly goals. Ask the Holy Spirit to help you live in line with His perfect goals for your weight loss and your life.

_____

_____

_____

_____

_____

_____

Day 2: Thurs

PRAYER FOR SACRIFICIAL LIVING

Devotion:

Today you will pray for a spirit that is willing to make sacrifices. Sadly, many of us are not willing to do what it takes to reach our health and weight loss goals. It's not because we're lazy or undeserving of having all we desire. It's because we don't understand the significance of short-term sacrifice for long-term gain. When we understand how much God truly loves us, we will see that sacrificing is more than just resisting a cookie or 10. Foregoing immediate gratification draws us to the true heart of God by removing all of the strongholds that keep us from knowing Him.

Focus your prayers today on discovering how to see sacrifice as a form of worship to God (Romans 12:1); as an opportunity to draw closer to God (James 4:8); as a way to strengthen our body, mind and spirit, and God's way of saving us from our destructive selves (James 1:14-15). Freedom is found in dying to ourselves every hour of every day so that we can live an abundant life.

The power to sacrifice does not come from your willpower or hard work. Rather, it's a natural response that comes from seeing God as He truly is—one who overwhelmingly and stead-fastly loves us.

Action:

Pray for a willing spirit of sacrifice.

Validation:

"God, You have given me the knowledge and tools for a healthful lifestyle, and I am grateful. I pray to not be tempt-ed and stay in my boundaries. Most of the time I am okay, but temptation is always there. I pray for the willingness to over-come (still) late-night treats."

"I am becoming aware of the difference between knowing the truth and experiencing the truth. I know God is better at comforting me than food, and that He deserves complete obe-dience and surrender. Yet, how often do I live this way? Time to live what I believe. For today, I pray I turn to God to settle me and comfort me. I also pray I remember it is an offense to choose self and short-term pleasure over obedience."

"I believe at the root of my fears of sacrificial living is loss. I'm afraid of losing things that I love whether that be food, re-lationships with people, time with people, the feeling of fitting in... I don't want to miss out on anything by denying myself anything. My reminder is that God is enough and I don't have to fill myself with anything or anyone other than Him."

Meditation:

Then Jesus said to his disciples, *"Whoever wants to be my disciple must deny themselves and take up their cross and follow me."* (Matthew 16:24)

Inspiration:

Great achievement is usually born of great sacrifice,
and is never the result of selfishness.
~ Napoleon Hill

Declaration:

I am as bold as a lion. I can endure to the end because You are my strength and shield. I have the capacity for victorious living. I operate in excellence and purpose to complete every task that I set out to do. I can do all things through Christ Who gives me strength. There is no temptation that can overtake me because You give me the strength to bear up under it. My sacrifice is my form of worship to You, so I do it with peace and gratitude.

Supplication:

Lord, You have given me the power and strength to develop a healthier lifestyle that glorifies You. Teach me how to give up my own unhealthy desires in order to glorify You and my body. I can endure the temptations because You are my strength and my shield. I can spend time planning to eat healthfully and exercise because You have given me the capacity for victorious living. I find complete healing in You! Thank You, Lord, for blessing me in every way! Amen!!

Reflection:

1. Take time to acknowledge your refusal to sacrifice certain foods, your time, or other things that God has called you to in order to be healthy. What do you refuse to sacrifice?

_____

_____

_____

_____

_____

_____

_____

_____

2. Now acknowledge the fears you have around sacrificing. Allow the Holy Spirit to show you what is at the root of those fears.

"Search me, God, and know my heart; test me and know my anxious thoughts."
(Psalm 139:233)

"Therefore, I urge you, brothers and sisters, in view of God's mercy, to offer your bodies as a living sacrifice, holy and pleasing to God—this is your true and proper worship."
(Romans 12:1)

_____

_____

_____

_____

_____

_____

3. In light of God's love for you and your love for Him, how will you offer your body as a living sacrifice as stated in scripture?

_____

_____

_____

_____

_____

_____

Day 3:

PRAYER FOR ACTION

Devotion:

Today you're going to pray for a willingness to take action on the habits you want to master. Too often we look back at the things we didn't do with regret. "If only I had stuck to my plan. If only I did it when I had the chance. I wish I had not eaten that." So much of our health journey and even our entire life is filled with regrets. It's time to pray against this spirit of regret.

That's not how our loving Heavenly Father designed us. Just think back to your childhood days in the playground. You dreamed of becoming a princess or superhero. No one ever dreams of living a life full of regrets and disappointments. Where did it all go awry?

Somewhere along the line, we lost touch with who we are in Christ and how much He truly loves us. Or maybe we never accepted this message. When we can truly grasp the depth of His love for us, then we can begin to live in faithfulness to whatever He has called us to—no regrets. When you bring this before God in prayer, you will begin living a life without regrets. As you spend time with Him, you'll develop an understanding of your worth, your value and your purpose in God, which will inspire you to take action.

Action:

Pray for courage to take action on the habits you want to master.

Validation:

"God is nudging me to keep reaching out to Him more often throughout each day. Reminders to commit my actions to Him (Prov. 16:3), and that in Him I live and move and have my being (Acts 17:28), are posted on my computer. God wants me to be the living sacrifice He calls me to be, and He is patient and loving and kind as He continues His good work in me."

"I believe as I obey God's call to stop impulsive eating I will enjoy confidence, joy, and peace. The pull of food will lessen, and I can enjoy freedom and enjoy my life more."

"God's plan for me is filling me completely with His promises of peace and His satisfaction with me as I am. God has taken my regrets from me. We are winning in this weight loss journey."

Meditation:

"If you keep quiet at a time like this, deliverance and relief for the Jews will arise from some other place, but you and our relatives will die."
(Esther 4:14 NLT)

Inspiration:

In the end, we only regret the chances we did not
take, the relationships we were afraid to have, and
the decisions we waited too long to make.
~ Lewis Carroll

Declaration:

All things work together for good. My pain will turn into laughter, my cross will be exchanged for a crown, and my mourning will be turned into dancing. I am blessed and I am a blessing. My disappointments of the past will be turned into testimonies, in the Name of Jesus.

Supplication:

Dear Lord, I pray that I would not sit idly by in the comfort of overeating and not exercising. You've shown me that the price is too high to pay. Lord, You have given me a vision for what my life will be like when I am totally surrendered to You and I am at a healthy weight, and the costs involved if I don't. I choose the better way. Strengthen my mind and will, Lord. In Your Name I pray. Amen!

Reflection:

1. Take a moment and reflect on the last time you experienced regret from sabotaging your health. Let God know that you choose His love, peace, and joy over your regrets. Allow Him to show you how the situation will be different the next time.

_____

_____

_____

_____

_____

_____

2. Take a moment right now and experience God's love. Let it fill your mind. Can you feel His pleasure? He is not mad at you. Read this scripture below as if your Heavenly Father is saying it to you right now.

> *"His master replied, 'Well done, good and faithful*
> *servant! You have been faithful with a few things;*
> *I will put you in charge of many things. Come and*
> *share your master's happiness!'"*
> (Matthew 25:23)

_____

_____

_____

_____

_____

_____

3. What good plans does God have for you today concerning your weight loss, so that you can experience His pleasure instead of your own regret?

_____

_____

_____

_____

_____

_____

_____

_____

_____

_____

_____

_____

_____

_____

Day 4:
Sat
PRAYER FOR PROGRESS

Devotion:

Today you're going to pray for understanding of the weight-releasing process—for wisdom, discernment, and peace.

Change takes time, patience, discipline, commitment, and a whole lot of grace. For example, if one night you break your boundaries and eat after 7:00 pm, when you said you wouldn't, don't beat up on yourself and sabotage your entire plan. Pray, renew your mind, and keep on going—no guilt, no condemnation, no shame—just keep on going. Too many of us think that because we set a goal, it should be smooth sailing without any setbacks, and then are distraught when setbacks come and quit altogether. Know that they WILL come and gird yourself up, so that you will continue on in victory from glory to glory.

We would much rather get to the end and bypass all of the ups and downs in the middle, but that would never draw us closer to God. Without going through the process, you will miss all the wonderful things your Heavenly Father wants to teach you and how He wants to strengthen you. Every time you grow weary, pray that you would stay the course and that you will not grow faint.

Action:

Think about the process and your progress as you pray to-day. Pray that you will embrace the process regardless of the pace.

Validation:

"It would take one year to lose 50 pounds at a rate of about 1 lb. per week! I would be thrilled to be 50 lbs. lighter this time next year!! I would look and feel great!"

"It will take me six months to attain my goal weight. I trust God to give me the strength and the resolve to keep moving forward."

"To get to a healthy weight, it will take one to two years. I am taking into account that I don't seem to drop weight as eas-ily. I would like to just be at a safe weight for me. 135-140 would be ideal, but as long as I am moving toward better health... That's all I want to focus on, better health."

Meditation:

"Little by little I will drive them out before you,
until you have increased enough to take possession
of the land."
(Exodus 23:30 NIV)

Inspiration:

"Take the first step in faith. You don't have to see the whole staircase, just take the first step."
~ Martin Luther King Jr.

"It's about progress, not perfection."
~ Unknown

Declaration:

Thank You for Your promises. I am making progress. From victory to victory, success to success, I am getting stronger each day. I am more than an overcomer. I am unstoppable and I am advancing in everything I put my mind to. I am unstoppable!

Supplication:

Dear Lord, some days the progress feels so slow and seems like it will take forever to reach a healthy weight. Thank you for reminding me that the process and its lessons are just as important as the progress. I am getting stronger and stronger each day. I am learning new things about You and myself each day, and I am more than an overcomer. I have victory in You, Lord! Thank You for your love, grace, and blessings! Amen!

Reflection:

1. Meditate on God's desire for you to stay the course, despite the highs and lows.

"Consider it all joy, my brethren, when you encounter various trials, knowing that the testing of your faith produces endurance. And let endurance have its perfect result, so that you may be perfect and complete, lacking in nothing..."
(James 1:3-4)

_____

_____

_____

_____

_____

_____

2. Ask God to lead you to some practical steps to get you through the next time you experience a low in your journey. What scriptures is He leading you to?

_____

_____

_____

_____

_____

_____

3. Ask God for the strength and perseverance to rise to worship Him in the highs and draw closer to Him during the low periods of your weight loss journey.

_____

_____

_____

_____

_____

_____

_____

_____

_____

_____

_____

_____

_____

_____

Day 5:
Sun

PRAYER OF SUBMISSION

Devotion:

Pray for the spirit of submission, that you will be led by the Spirit and not by your flesh.

The concept of submission has been marred by the world, but when we look at it in light of God's love for us we see a very different picture. Imagine a picture of a loving, gentle, patient yet strong father who cares for our every need and promises us rest, joy, peace, and protection if we will abide in Him and Him alone.

He knows that those diet pills, the surgeries, or the latest 'how to lose weight' book will never satisfy that longing to fix the feelings of unworthiness in ourselves. Submitting our will to Him is the only way to health, healing, and wholeness. That's how much He loves us.

It's time to stop trying to achieve your goals on your own terms. How much more money will you spend? How much more time will you waste? How many more days of frustration will you experience? Listen, if you could have done it on your own you would have already done it. Give it to God, and believe that He is more than able to do for you what you can't do for your-self.

Action:

Pray for the spirit of submission. Pray that you will be led by the Spirit and not by your own flesh.

Validation:

"I've never seriously involved God in my weight loss (1st time)... so I need to seriously involve God in this journey... submit it to Him. Secondly, I need to do it through prayer and studying scriptures."

"Like many others have said, I have trouble giving up control. We are taught that you get good results by working hard and you can only rely on yourself. I know God will expect me to work hard at this, but I also know I will only be truly successful at becoming more healthy if I keep my focus on Him, keep my priorities straight, and rely on Him by being in Scripture and prayer. By trusting Him for guidance and strength, I should actually reduce my stress by knowing HE has control! This is hard for me—I'm kind of a control-freak, but will keep asking Him to help me give it to Him every morning."

"I believe I need to submit my fear of being smaller. My weight has always been my shield. My thought is I will no longer have my weight to hide behind. I am being led to restart writing in my journal and to not miss a morning reading my word. At one time I was very faithful with my journaling and reading my YouVersion devotions. I need to make a more concentrated effort to be consistent with both."

Meditation:

"The LORD went before them by day in a pillar of cloud to lead them along the way, and by night in a pillar of fire to give them light."
(Exodus13:21-22 ESV)

Inspiration:

"Forgive me for picking up what I already laid at your feet."
~ Unknown

"Prayer is not about letting God know your will; it's about completely submitting to Him. You die to yourself."
~ Mark Batterson

Declaration:

I walk in Your presence today and I choose to honor You, God, by what I eat, and in all I do. I submit my weight, my health, and my body to You. I walk with courage, discipline, and perseverance in times of testing and temptation. I am blessed and prosperous in You.

Supplication:

Dear Lord, I come to You humbly and admit to You that I can't release this unhealthy weight on my own. I've tried for so long and in so many different ways. Lord, I open my heart and mind to Your prompting as I submit to You. I invite You to lead me in this process; I commit to do Your will. In Your Name I pray. Amen!

Reflection:

1. Author Charles Swindoll says,

"The problem with a living sacrifice is that it keeps crawling off the altar". What aspect of your health journey do you have to continually keep placing back on the altar?

Not eating at night

_____

_____

_____

_____

_____

_____

_____

2. Reflect on how much God loves you. His desire is that we would tangibly experience His love as we spend time with Him.

"We love because he first loved us."
(1 John 4:19)

*"So we have come to know and to believe the love
that God has for us. God is love, and whoever abides
in love abides in God, and God abides in him."*
(1 John 4:16)

_____

_____

_____

_____

_____

_____

3. Allow the Holy Spirit to lead you to a life of submission today. Let Him renew you with a fresh perspective on submission, and with strength to stop taking back what you keep submitting.

_____

_____

_____

_____

_____

Day 6:
_M on_

PRAYER FOR GOD'S PRESENCE

Devotion:

Today you're going to pray for the conviction to turn every worry, concern, and complaint into a conversation with God.

Have you been complaining about your weight for years? Then guess what? You know how to pray! Take the same effort and energy that you've been using to talk about your weight and simply turn it upside down.

Instead of complaining about it, ask God what HIS will is for you in the area of your health and LISTEN for his response. He WILL show you what to do. Spend time in prayer listening for the heartbeat of God, and let His love for you and the knowledge of His will transform all of your worries to a heart of worship, praise, and accompanying peace. That's the power of prayer, and that's the power of God's love for us.

Action:

Pray for the conviction to turn every worry, concern, and complaint into a conversation with God.

Validation:

"Dear Lord, You know my innermost being and You know deep down what the root cause of my overeating is. I pray that You would reveal that to me, and that You would bring healing to those areas of my life. Lord, I want to glorify You with my whole being, and right now I'm not. I want to put food in its rightful place and You above all else! Guide me, Holy Spirit, and show me the way. Lord, I submit myself and this journey to You. In Jesus' Name I pray. Amen!"

"Father God, the desire of my heart is to live in obedience to You and Your plan for my life. I believe that part of that plan is to live a healthy lifestyle. So I ask You to help me do this today with my eating. I ask that the Holy Spirit remind me of this as we spend time with family at the zoo and enjoy the lunch that will be provided for us. In Jesus' Name, Amen."

"Father God, You know I have walked this road of weight loss many times before and have generally not been successful and not been disciplined to stick to it long enough. This time is different, Father. I submit this journey to You, each and every moment of every day. I pray that I will stop idolizing food and obsessing over it all the time. I know that with Your help and me allowing your involvement in this food walk, I can be disciplined to lose this weight. Thank You that you want to be included in every aspect of my life. Thank You for loving me the way I am. May I learn to love myself inside and out, too. Amen xx."

"Pray that you will not fall into temptation."
(Luke 22:40)

Inspiration:

> *"A Bible that's falling apart usually belongs to someone who isn't."*
> ~ Charles Spurgeon

Declaration:

I thank You that we don't have to be worried or anxious about anything. We bring our request to You with thanksgiving and stand in confidence that You will bring it to fruition. We submit our request to You and are able to do exceedingly, abundantly, above all that we can ask or think.

Supplication:

Dear Lord, it is such a comfort to know that You are always right there! All I need to do is just start talking to You and You listen with such love and compassion. I need You, Lord, now more than ever. These patterns of unhealthy eating and not exercising are so ingrained in me. I need Your healing touch in my life. I need Your guidance. Lord, I want to be a blessing to You and glorify You in my body. Thank You that I don't need to fret over how this will transpire; You have this all under control, and I submit myself to You. In Your Name I pray. Amen!

Reflection:

1. Reflect on why you don't always go to God in prayer. Is it because you tried it in the past and it didn't work? Maybe you can believe it for other people but not for yourself. Or because

you've never given it a fair try. Whatever your reason, let God know your true desire to become a person of prayer, and listen for how He responds to your request.

> "The heartfelt and persistent prayer of a righteous man (believer) can accomplish much [when put into action and made effective by God—it is dynamic and can have tremendous power]."
> (James 5:16b AMP)

_____

_____

_____

_____

_____

_____

_____

2. The Bible teaches us that faith comes from hearing the Word of God. What scripture is the Holy Spirit leading you to that will strengthen your faith?

> "And whatever you ask in prayer, you will receive, if you have faith."
> (Matthew 21:22)

*"So faith comes from hearing, and hearing through
the word of Christ."*
(Romans 10:17)

_____

_____

_____

_____

_____

_____

_____

3. Ask the Holy Spirit to help you turn all of your complaints about your weight into prayers that God can hear and transform in you (mind, soul, spirit).

_____

_____

_____

_____

_____

_____

_____

Day 7: Tues

PRAYER FOR MAKING RIGHT CHOICES

Devotion:

It seems crazy that, given the choice of light or darkness, good or bad, right or wrong, action or slothfulness, and nutritious foods over junk, we continually choose the latter. Why? We know it's not right for us, yet we can't seem to help ourselves. That's why we should never make any decisions on our own without the power of the Holy Spirit. You have a choice to meet with God, read His Word, and spend time allowing Him to mold your actions and decisions. Know that when you choose God, His power will transform your darkness into light, your bad into good, your wrong into right, and your slothfulness into action. The choice is yours today.

Action:

Pray for the strength, courage, and conviction to make good choices today that will positively impact your weight loss.

Validation:

"Lord, Your Word says in Philippians 4:13 that I can do ALL things through You who strengthens me. I choose to develop more strongly the habit to come to You for strength before I eat anything, so I may eat healthfully and in the right portions. Thank You for Your faithfulness."

"Heavenly Father, thank You that You are intimately involved in my weight loss. Your Word says that all things are permissible, but not all things are beneficial. I pray for help to choose that which is beneficial in this very moment. Teach me to be satisfied with what fuels my body instead of what feeds my flesh. All praise and glory to You. In Your Name I pray. Amen."

"Deuteronomy 30:18-20: 'This day I call the heavens and the earth as witnesses against you, that I have set before you life and death, blessings and curses. Now choose life, so that you and your children may live and that you may love the Lord your God, listen to his voice, and hold fast to him.' Lord, let me choose life, each moment, each meal, each temptation. I choose life, because I choose to follow You!"

Meditation:

"This day I call the heavens and the earth as witnesses against you that I have set before you life and death, blessings and curses. Now choose life, so that you and your children may live."
(Deuteronomy 30:19 NIV)

Inspiration:

> *"You are free to make whatever choice you want, but you are not free from the consequences of the choice."*
> ~ Unknown

Declaration:

I am dead to sin. Your strength and grace have changed me and renewed me. I have a new life in You, and do things that lead to holiness and joy. The power of Your life-giving Spirit has freed me from the power of sin. Your Spirit that controls my mind has given me life and peace.

Supplication:

Dear Lord, thank You that I am a new creation in You. I pray that my mind and heart would grasp this, and that I would rest in Your amazing transforming power and love. Lord, please reveal to me what small step You would have me take to make a healthy change in my life. I get so overwhelmed when I try to do it in my own strength, so I'm giving this all to You. I also turn discouragement and fear over to You right now and claim the power I have in You. I can do all things through You, because You give me strength! Amen

Reflection:

1. Reflect on the choices you made at your last meal. Do they foster life or death? If they foster the latter, ask yourself what

you can to do make a better choice the next time you are in a similar situation.

_____

_____

_____

_____

_____

_____

_____

2. Ask the Holy Spirit to help you with the ability to make good choices today.

_____

_____

_____

_____

_____

_____

3. Pray in accordance with what the Holy Spirit is showing you about the choices you make around your weight loss. What scriptures are you being led to that will minister to you when you need to make decisions in this area?

_____

_____

_____

_____

_____

_____

_____

_____

_____

_____

_____

_____

_____

_____

_____

[handwritten note: Make a U Turn to things you don't need!]

Day 8:
Wed

PRAYER FOR SPEAKING LIFE OVER YOURSELF

Devotion:

Beautiful, lovely, breathtaking, gorgeous, awesome, pretty, at-tractive, inspiring, powerful, inspirational, amazing, success-ful, accomplished, trail-blazing—most of us would have no trouble attributing many of these qualities to famous women we see on TV or read about, but what about you? Can you at-tribute these qualities to yourself? They're all in you, too! God loved you so much that He created you in His image. So look in the mirror and begin to speak life into yourself. You are all these things and more!

Speaking life is critical for your weight loss journey. If you don't feel worthy of having a healthy body, then you will con-tinue to repel the very things you say you want. Change starts in the mind and is reflected by your actions.

Action:

Today, you will pray that you would use your tongue to af-firm and bless yourself and the wonder that you are. You will speak life over yourself; you will speak blessings!

Validation:

"Oh, those negative comments I make in the mirror of my bathroom. I fail to see the beauty and the glow that God has given me. But today I thank Him for the Temple He has given me and the work He is doing to restore my body and my soul. He has given me the strength to run and not be weary, walk and not faint. Lord, I thank you!"

"I tend to get negative about my stomach. I'll say "how did this happen? I feel fat". God loves me as I am. He loves me so much He's helping me to change. This belly will be a normal size before long. I'm fearfully and wonderfully made. God is doing a work inside and out!"

"I have a terrible problem with negative talk about myself. Not only in how I look, but the mother I was when my kids were younger, the mother I am now. I could be a better friend, co-worker... the list goes on. When I start the negative thinking, I have started to turn to God and remind myself I am made in His image and He loves me. I love my family and friends, and I have done the best I could, and can."

Meditation:

"The tongue has the power of life and death."
(Proverbs 18:21 NIV)

Inspiration:

The greatest discovery of my generation is that human beings can alter their lives by altering their attitudes of mind.
~ William James

Declaration:

I have the faith to move mountains. The Holy Spirit in me has made the impossible possible. I am more than a conqueror, and I can overcome any obstacle that stands in my path. No weapon formed against me shall prosper. I am constantly making progress. I am a success.

Supplication:

Dear Lord, I am strong and courageous because of You. I am fearfully and wonderfully made! So Lord, I am boldly asking in faith to be an overcomer in the areas I struggle with in my life, especially with food, exercise, and negative self-talk. I pray that You would help me to see myself as you see me. Although my faith is as small as a mustard seed, You say in Your Word that it is enough to move a mountain! In You and through You I am making progress. May I bring You glory as people see the changes in my life. Thank You for coming alongside me and being my rock! I ask these things in the powerful Name of Jesus. Amen!

Reflection:

1. Meditate on what the Bible says about the power of your words.

> "It is not what goes into the mouth that defiles
> a person, but what comes out of the mouth;
> this defiles a person."
> (Matthew 15:11)

> *"We demolish arguments and every pretension that sets itself up against the knowledge of God, and we take captive every thought to make it obedient to Christ."*
> (2 Corinthians 10:5)

I don't know how to handle this but you do God.

_____

_____

_____

_____

_____

2. Ask God what He thinks of you. Then make a list as long as you can of all the attributes that He says about you.

_____

_____

_____

_____

_____

_____

3. As you go about your day today, ask the Holy Spirit to help you notice your negative speech (and thoughts) and replace it with something affirming.

_____

_____

_____

_____

_____

_____

_____

_____

_____

_____

_____

_____

_____

_____

_____

Day 9:

Ihus

PRAYER FOR CONSCIOUS LIVING

Devotion:

Today you will pray that you will experience God's presence at all times as you move throughout the day.

Most of us never take the time to think about what we're thinking about. If we were to tune in to our thoughts, we would realize so much about ourselves. We would realize that we're either worrying about things in the past (I wish I had exercised yesterday, or I should not have eaten that cake), or we're worried about the future (I've got to get to the gym, or I've got to get my eating under control).

Yet, the place where we're most powerful and effective is the one place we spend the least amount of time, and that's in the here and now—the present—where God is. He is here right now and He wants to meet with you here. Will you focus on this present moment and fellowship with Him? The more you can focus on Him, the more the cares of this world will fade away.

Action:

Pray that you would experience God's presence at all times.

Validation:

"I'm much more aware of everything that I'm eating now. Before, I would just eat whatever would satisfy me. Boy, does that make a difference, especially when I'm incorporating 10,000 steps a day. I don't want all of that effort to be in vain."

"Went out to dinner last night for my husband's birthday. Did really good at the dinner. Passed up the rolls. Had kabobs with grilled veggies, green beans, and salad. Felt good about it, then sabotaged myself by staying up too late, getting really hungry, and caved by eating chocolate chip cookies. Failed to have planned snacks on hand, but more importantly staying up too late always gets me into trouble. Or maybe it's closet eating when everyone goes to bed."

"For breakfast I had two eggs and fruit. That is my usual breakfast. I need the protein and enjoy the fruit. Lunch was a salmon fillet, brown and wild rice, Brussels sprouts in a light butter sauce, and two dried natural figs. I am feeling great about my choices and have lots of energy."

Meditation:

"Where can I go from your Spirit? Or where can I flee from your presence?"
(Psalm 139:7 NIV)

Inspiration:

"Let us not look back in anger, nor forward in fear,
but around in awareness."
~ James Thurber

Declaration:

I love You, Lord, and thank You for Your Spirit that lives in me. My mind is set on things above. I become more and more like You each day. I am created in Your image. I make responsible choices and decisions. I have the ability to solve my problems with You as my guide. I take authority over this day, in the Name of Jesus.

Supplication:

Dear Lord, I choose to live consciously in the here and now. I will check in with You hour by hour and trust that You will show me how to be more aware of my eating patterns. I am being transformed and renewed day by day by living my life in You and by keeping my mind set on things above. I pray, Lord, for continued strength to make wise decisions regarding my weight loss. I know I can do all things through You, and by Your grace I am becoming more and more like You every day. In Your Name I pray. Amen!

Reflection:

1. Meditate on what the Bible says about God's constant presence in your life.

"Where shall I go from your Spirit? Or where shall I flee from your presence? If I ascend to heaven, you are there! If I make my bed in Sheol, you are there! If I take the wings of the morning and dwell in the uttermost parts of the sea, even there your hand shall lead me, and your right hand shall hold me."
(Psalm 139:7-10)

"Fear not, for I have redeemed you; I have called you by name, you are mine. When you pass through the waters, I will be with you; and through the rivers, they shall not overwhelm you; when you walk through fire you shall not be burned, and the flame shall not consume you. For I am the Lord your God, the Holy One of Israel, your Savior."
(Isaiah 43:1-3)

_____

_____

_____

_____

_____

_____

_____

_____

_____

2. Close your eyes right now and tune in to God's presence. What feelings do you experience? What do you hear God telling you? What do you see?

_____

_____

_____

_____

_____

_____

_____

_____

_____

3. Whether you can feel him or not, God is here and He is with you right now. Ask Him to fill you with His presence. Ask the Holy Spirit to help you remain in the present whenever your mind reverts back to the past or races ahead of God into the future.

Day 10:
THE PRAYER OF THE INSIGHT

Devotion:

Today, pray for insight into your life from God's perspective instead of from your own view.

Sadly, many of us spend much of our lives frustrated with ourselves. We constantly beat up on ourselves for continually making the same mistakes over and over, and can never seem to gain any traction. It's because true insight about ourselves, our bodies, and our health, only comes about when we learn who we are in Christ.

Insight is important because it helps us control our eternal destiny. It's impossible to leave a lasting impact in this world if we do not feel in control of our thoughts or our actions—like they are always holding us captive. If we can't use our God-given power to keep ourselves from eating a piece of chocolate, how confident are we that we can take charge of our God-given destiny?

When we spend time in prayer, God alone can teach us why we do what we do and why we continually spin our wheels or sabotage ourselves. He will give you insight into yourself and show you just how significant, powerful, and purposeful you are. He longs to show you your life from His perspective if you will allow Him. God yearns for us to gain insight and see through the lens of the Holy Spirit and His Word—that's where our breakthrough will come.

Action:

Pray for insight into your life from His perspective instead of from your own view.

Validation:

"I don't believe I can change...I have been a big girl all my life, loving to eat!"

"I think, 'Why can everybody else eat that and I can't? That's not fair!'"

"I am afraid that if I start a diet, I will go back to thinking that when I am skinny, people will like me, love me more...so that is what stops me."

"My problem is excuse-making and blaming. I usually end up eating un-nutritious foods when my friends are around, telling myself that it's just this one time...I also end up making excuses for not working out and they are usually things that are super insignificant like, it's too hot out, when I know hot weather is what I love to work out in."

"The two biggest for me from childhood to now (65), always have seemed to be emotional eating and self-esteem issues. I grew up in an alcoholic and food-addicted family, and it is difficult to move beyond some of the issues deeply embedded. But honestly, just loving the taste of food and its effects is a lot of it for me, too."

Meditation:

"I do not understand what I do. For what
I want to do I do not do, but what I hate I do."
(Romans 7:15 NIV)

Inspiration:

"Character is expressed through our behavior
patterns, or natural responses to things."
~ Joyce Meyer

Declaration:

Have mercy on me, Christ. You have searched me, God, and helped me uncover my anxious thoughts. I now begin the process of rooting them out forever. I thank You for replacing my old behaviors with new ones that are pleasing in Your eyes. Because of Your love I am dead to sin. I boldly take hold of Your power that gives me victory over sin.

Supplication:

Dear Lord, I do what I do not want to do and don't do what I want to do, but that is because I am trying to do this in my own power. Lord, I submit my recurring patterns to You. I submit my whole life to You. Your ways are so much better than mine. Help me come to grips with my sinful nature so that I may abide in You fully. Replace my fears and faults with Christ's freedom— You are the only one who can give true lasting victory from the bondage of un-nutritious eating and lack of exercising. I want to glorify You, Lord, with my life! Amen!

Reflection:

1. Only God can help you understand yourself in this world where we've lost our way due to past circumstances, worry, doubt, fear, and insecurity. Meditate on what His Word says about how we are to live.

"The world is passing away along with its desires, but whoever does the will of God abides forever."
(1 John 2:17)

"Do not lay up for yourselves treasures on earth, where moth and rust destroy and where thieves break in and steal, but lay up for yourselves treasures in heaven, where neither moth nor rust destroys and where thieves do not break in and steal. For where your treasure is, there your heart will be also."
(Matthew 6:19-21)

_____

_____

_____

_____

_____

2. Reflect on your own life.

How much of your time is spent trying to fix yourself? How many self-help books, courses, and programs have you tried in order to gain insight into your destructive habit? God wants to give you insight into all these areas. Invite Him in today.

> *"Search me, O God, and know my heart;*
> *Try me and know my anxious thoughts;*
> *And see if there be any hurtful way in me,*
> *And lead me in the everlasting way."*
> (Psalm 129:23-24)

_____

_____

_____

_____

_____

_____

_____

_____

_____

_____

3. Repent for always trying to find the answers on your own. Tell God that you trust His will and His way, and you want only His insight and wisdom for your life.

_____

_____

_____

_____

_____

_____

_____

_____

_____

_____

_____

_____

_____

_____

Day 11:
Sat

PRAYER TO OVERCOME LIMITING BELIEFS

Devotion:

Today, pray for insight into your limiting beliefs and that they will no longer hold you captive.

Two of the worst effects sin has on us as Christian women are that it distorts our view about who we really are in Christ, and as a result we create limiting beliefs that keep us from becoming who Christ has called us to be.

Limiting beliefs are lies or false beliefs that we have about ourselves that developed as a result of what was said to us in our childhood or how we interpreted something that was said to us (e.g., you'll never amount to anything; you're useless; you're not wanted, etc.).

If we formed limiting beliefs about God, we can believe that God is angry with us, that He is judging us, or that we are not worthy of His love when we don't take care of our bodies as we should. The truth is that God is not mad at you. He desires today that you would come to see yourself as he does—without spot or blemish (Eph 5:27). And that your limiting beliefs will no longer impact your memory, your thoughts, your habits, and your identity; and that lies will no longer separate you from His love. Christ did that for us on the cross, and our assignment is to draw close to Him and His truths.

Active:

Pray that your limiting beliefs will no longer hold you captive.

Validation:

"I think one of my limiting beliefs was feeling that I didn't quite measure up. This kept me working harder to be successful, and in many ways I was successful, but I was also anxious. And as I have said before, food was always a way that I could feel better. The thing that is helping me the most is becoming aware of God's great and all-encompassing love for me."

"My limited belief is you live once, might as well enjoy it."

"I have belief that I won't be happy if I don't eat what I want and when I want. And I am thinking also that I am afraid to lose weight, as I am afraid will anyone want to date me or even get to know me if my personality also changes traumatically. These are lies not truth. I know I will be healthier thinner, and more energetic, and I believe also much happier. And change is sometimes for good."

Meditation:

"...They continued to follow their own gods
according to the religious customs of the nations
from which they came."
(2 Kings 17:33 NLT)

Inspiration:

*"Growth demands a temporary surrender of security.
It may mean giving up familiar but limiting patterns,
safe but unrewarding work, values no longer believed
in, and relationships that have lost their meaning."*
~ John C. Maxwell

Declaration:

Your promises are for eternity. Every generational curse and everything spoken against my health is broken in the Name of Jesus. I declare that I am in sound health in my body, mind, and spirit. I am strong and courageous, and successful in everything I do. I meditate on Your Word day and night. Him who the Son sets free is free indeed, and I declare my freedom in You.

Supplication:

Dear Lord, I pray that in Your mighty power You would break every generational curse and everything spoken against my weight loss. Lord, You want healing and wholeness in my life and I can't do this in my own strength, so I lay my life and its brokenness at the foot of Your cross. I declare victory in You. I am strong and courageous and successful in all that I do because You promise that those who the Son sets free are free indeed! In Your Name I pray. Amen!

Reflection:

1. Meditate on what the Bible says about God's desire to heal you of your limiting beliefs. *"But he said to me, 'My grace is suffi-cient for you, for my power is made perfect in weakness.' Therefore I*

will boast all the more gladly of my weaknesses, so that the power of Christ may rest upon me." (2 Corinthians 12:9)

_____

_____

_____

_____

_____

_____

_____

_____

"The LORD is near to the brokenhearted.
And saves those who are crushed in spirit."
(Psalm 34:18)

2. Ask the Holy Spirit to show you some limiting beliefs you have about God, His sovereignty, and His ability to meet all of your needs.

_____

_____

_____

_____

_____

3. Spend some time in prayer and allow God to exchange your limiting beliefs for His truths. What truths is He showing you about yourself and who He is in your life?

_____

_____

_____

_____

_____

_____

_____

_____

_____

_____

_____

_____

_____

_____

Day 12:
PRAYER TO OVERCOME EXCUSES

Devotion:

Today, pray that you would notice when you're making excuses and learn to take responsibility for your actions.

We're so quick to come up with a reason for why we don't do what we said we were going to do. It often seems like we would rather produce reasons instead of getting results. Why are we excuse-making machines? I ate this because ... I did not exercise because ...

As long as we have a reason for why we did not do what we set out to do, we will never achieve our results. It's because we don't want to admit to ourselves that we did not do what we said we would do, and it's easier to blame extenuating circumstances instead of accepting responsibility for our own actions or inaction.

What God requires from us is honesty more than anything. Commit to turning all of your excuses and reasons over to God. That's the only way we can learn to overcome them. It's only when we allow the Holy Spirit to work at the core of our being and transform us from the inside out that we can begin to produce results instead of reasons.

Action:

Pray that you would notice when you're making excuses, and learn to take responsibility for your actions.

Validation:

"I get so busy with work and home responsibilities. I'm too mentally tired to focus on all this."

READ LUKE 10:38-42 (Mary and Martha).

"I am older and more tired. It's too late (in life) to deal with these things."

READ HEBREWS 11. Notice all the older individuals with the faith they had to accomplish what God asked them to do.

"It's in my genes to struggle with weight; I've had four kids—it's gonna look like it; all that healthy food is expensive; I don't have time for all the praying that this would require; I've worked hard all week so I deserve a day off; it's too hard to plan meals when I'm traveling or eating out; I have a thyroid condition that makes it very hard to lose weight."

And my Lord's answer?

2 Corinthians 12:9

"...but He said to me, 'My grace is sufficient for you, for My strength is made perfect in weakness.'"

"One of my biggest excuses for not walking is 'I'm too tired, I didn't sleep well last night'. And while it is true that I often don't sleep well, I am going to be tired whether I walk or not, and frequently after I walk I actually feel better."

My scripture for this excuse is Philippians 4:13. *"I can do all things through Christ which strengthens me."*

Another excuse is: "You've done this before. You are initially successful then you stop following the program. What is the use of ailing again."

My scripture for that excuse is Deuteronomy 2:3 NASB: *"You've circled this mountain long enough."* Also, Proverbs 24:16.

Meditation:

"I have no one to help me into the pool when the water is stirred. While I am trying to get in, someone else goes down ahead of me."
(John 5:7 NIV)

Inspiration:

"He that is good for making excuses is seldom good for anything else."
~ Benjamin Franklin

"If you really want to do something, you'll find a way. If you don't, you'll find an excuse."
~ Jim Rohn

Declaration:

Father, You've clothed me with strength and honor; You've empowered me to be strong and courageous. I reclaim my power in You by taking 100% responsibility for my thoughts and actions. I am blessed with the Holy Ghost to accomplish my weight-loss goals. I will have a testimony, in the Name of Jesus.

Supplication:

Dear Lord, I have made excuses long enough. Yes Lord, I want to get well! Show me what excuses are holding me back from glorifying You in my body, even ones I hold on to subconsciously. You have empowered me with Your Holy Spirit and I claim that power and will take 100% responsibility for my thoughts and actions so that I will accomplish my goal of getting to a healthy weight. In Your Name I pray. Amen!

Reflection:

1. Meditate on what the Bible says about taking responsibility.

> *"Arise, for it is your task, and we are with you;*
> *be strong and do it."*
> (Ezra 10:4)

> *"For we must all appear before the judgment seat of Christ, so that each one may receive what is due for what he has done in the body, whether good or evil.*
> (2 Corinthians 5:10)

_____

_____

_____

_____

_____

_____

_____

_____

2. Ask the Holy Spirit to show you why you continually make excuses. What are some of the fears behind it? What is He show-ing you?

_____

_____

_____

_____

_____

_____

3. Repent for giving up, refusing to take responsibility for your life by making excuses, and ask the Holy Spirit to teach you how to change this habit. What will you do the next time you catch yourself making an excuse instead of taking care of your weight loss?

_____

_____

_____

_____

_____

_____

_____

_____

_____

_____

_____

_____

_____

_____

Day 13:
mon

PRAYER FOR OVERCOMING BLAMING

Today, pray for courage to take 100% responsibility for your weight loss journey when you find yourself wanting to blame others.

Many of us have very legitimate reasons for why we developed poor eating habits or why we're inactive. Many of us experienced abuse, abandonment, neglect, and shame at the hands of those who were supposed to care for us, and so we feel quite justified to cast blame. Except we're all grown up, and as adults we now have a responsibility to right the wrongs that were done to us.

Spending the rest of our lives blaming them will only keep us from receiving the love and peace that God has for us. Blaming them will keep the open wounds festering, and we will continue to feel the pain. So even though what happened to us was not our fault, as adults it's now our responsibility to learn from it and move on.

In a second scenario, you may have so many people dependent on you right now that you may also be consciously or subconsciously blaming them for your inability to move forward on your goals. In this case, practice healthy self-care before you can take care of them. This will be a win-win for everyone.

When we choose to take responsibility for all of our actions, we will experience satisfaction unknown to those who blame and make excuses. We will experience the joy and peace of God's covering that comes by doing His will—that's the power of self-responsibility.

Action:

Pray for courage to take 100% responsibility for your weight loss journey.

Validation:

"I blame, to a small degree, my mom and husband. It seems like when I'm really working hard to lose weight and eat in a nourishing way, they buy treats and things and offer them to me or, if it's my mom and we're driving, she'll just put it in my lap. I fully realize that I have a choice to eat it or not, but food has always been my mom's way of numbing herself and I've always been her partner. Even as young as four I have memories of donuts eaten with the caution: 'Don't tell Dad!' As far as hubby, he'll bring home things he knows I love and offer them, or just eat them in front of me, commenting on how they are so good. It's a bit frustrating to say the least!"

"Well, I have to confess God is on my list. I am sorry for blaming God for my sins. My heart is very heavy with this revealing today. I do repent of allowing this to remain in my thinking. In prayer I went through the past baggage and released everyone who came to mind. I thought I was done but couldn't come to close my prayer time. It was like the Holy Spirit was saying, 'You're not done'. I was holding on to blaming God—still in a spiral today."

"I moved in with my mom when my dad passed away to help take care of her. I always blamed her for not being able to lose weight because she loved the casseroles, meat and pota-toes, and all those fattening foods. My ex-husband use to say 'you can eat more than that.' And I was thinking about this the other day. When I have been at a good weight and in good shape (I have been up and down all my life with the weight problem), people would say to me, 'I hope you don't get fat.' Why would someone say that???"

Meditation:

"The man replied, 'It was the woman you gave me who gave me the fruit, and I ate it.'"
(Genesis 3:12)

"How long are you going to wait before taking possession of the remaining land the Lord, the God of your ancestors, has given to you?"
(Joshua 18:3 NLT)

Inspiration:

"I'm only going to stand before God and give an account for my life, not for somebody else's life. If I have a bad attitude, then I need to say there's no point in me blaming you for what's wrong in my life."
~ Joyce Meyer

Declaration:

Father, forgive me for usurping my responsibility to You for my weight loss and wellness. Excellent health is mine. Energy and vitality are mine. I am designed to reach higher levels of health from victory to victory, glory to glory, in the Name of Jesus!

Supplication:

Dear Lord, forgive me for playing the blame game. Thank You for revealing to me who and what I blame for my excess weight. I claim 100% responsibility right now! Forgive me for holding on to past hurts and faulty ideas. Lord, help me to forgive those I need to forgive and to let go of those past hurts and feelings that I have been holding on to for so long. Bring healing to those wounded areas of my heart. I claim excellent health and energy right now! In Your precious Name I pray. Amen!

Reflection:

1. Meditate on God's Word about self-responsibility. What do you need to do in light of studying His Word?

"For each will have to bear his own load."
(Galatians 6:5)

2. Ask the Holy Spirit to help you forgive those that you feel caused you to develop poor eating habits, poor exercise habits, poor self-esteem, or anything else that's keeping you from achieving optimal health.

"Whoever conceals his transgressions will not prosper, but he who confesses and forsakes them will obtain mercy."
(Proverbs 28:13)

_____

_____

_____

_____

_____

3. Ask the Holy Spirit to guide you in all of the areas where you have been blaming others for your poor health. Repent and commit to living a blameless life from now on.

_____

_____

_____

_____

Day 14:

Tues

PRAYER FOR OVERCOMING PROCRASTINATION

Devotion:

Today, pray to overcome the spirit of procrastination as you notice yourself putting off something that you need to do.

Ask yourself, "Why do I put off my exercise program? Why do I decide to start my healthy eating regimen tomorrow instead of right now?" I once heard someone say, very tongue-in-cheek, that tomorrow they would stop procrastinating. Sadly for her, and for many of us, tomorrow will never come until we learn that procrastination can only be stopped by taking immediate action.

Believe it or not, our procrastination is directly related to our level of trust in God. If we really trusted Him at His Word, then we would not hesitate. If we really believed what His Word says, then we would not worry about failing, losing control, getting overwhelmed, being judged, or any of the other fears that keep us procrastinating. I pray that you will take time and discover how trustworthy our Heavenly Father is. When you do that, you will be empowered to take action; not in your own strength, but in the strength and power of your loving Father.

Action:

Pray to overcome the spirit of procrastination.

Validation:

"I procrastinate on exercise. I know I need to do it and I will discuss it at length with myself, but I never do it. One reason I never do it is because tomorrow sounds better. That way, if I say tomorrow that means I'm still 'committed' and will do it. It allows me to put it off but not feel so guilty because, after all, I have full intentions to do it at a later time."

"I think I procrastinate the most with planning my meals and praying. Planning my meals because I fear not succeeding with it, and so often I have a gorgeous meal plan and life happens and it flies out the window."

"There are two things that I have been procrastinating on. Tracking–I can come up with a thousand excuses why I can't track what I just ate. And taking a moment to pray before I cave in to a temptation. Usually I cave first and then ask for forgiveness later. I think I procrastinate on these things because I'm afraid of what might happen if I actually follow through on them—I might have to continue to do it and then eventually I'll fail."

Meditation:

"How long are you going to wait before taking possession of the remaining land the Lord, the God of your ancestors, has given to you?"
(Joshua 18:3 NLT)

Inspiration:

*"Procrastination may relieve short-term pressure.
But it often impedes long-term progress."*
~ John Maxwell

Declaration:

I seek Your Kingdom above all else. I put You before my agendas, my time-lines, and my priorities. I walk in faith and not fear. I walk in power, victory, and a sound mind. I do everything on time and in order. All my steps are ordered by You.

Supplication:

Dear Lord, I want more of You and less of me. I put my priorities, time, and anything that I put before You aside. Lord, You know my fears and all that hinders me from totally surrendering to You. Reveal to me those things that I'm not even aware of, and convict me of my procrastinating. I don't want anything holding me back from moving forward in victory towards my goal of a healthy weight and healthy body, so I claim victory in Your Holy Name! You give me power and a sound mind in order to be an overcomer. In Your Name I pray. Amen!

Reflection:

1. Meditate on what the Bible says about procrastination. *"See then that ye walk circumspectly, not as fools, but as wise, Redeeming the time, because the days are evil. Wherefore be ye not un-*

wise, but understanding what the will of the Lord [is]." (Ephesians 5:15-17)

> *"In what ways do you lack trust in God's ability to do what He says? Ask the Holy Spirit to help you trust Him more for it is God who works in you to will and to act in order to fulfill his good purpose."*
> (Philippians 2:13)

> *"Let us hold unswervingly to the hope we profess, for he who promised is faithful."*
> (Hebrews 10:23)

_____

_____

_____

_____

_____

_____

2. Ask the Holy Spirit to show you what fears are at the root of why you procrastinate.

_____

_____

_____

_____

3. Submit all of those fears to God and let Him know that you trust Him to help you learn how to take action on everything He has called you to do.

_____

_____

_____

_____

_____

_____

_____

_____

_____

_____

_____

_____

_____

_____

Day 15:
wed

PRAYER FOR OVERCOMING EMOTIONAL EATING

Devotion:

Today, pray that your emotions will be brought under God's submission.

Do you ever feel like you are being held hostage by your emotions? What's even worse is that food is your default for whatever emotion you're experiencing. You're angry—you eat. You're tired—you eat. You're frustrated—you eat. You're happy—you eat. They dictate what type of day you will have, what you will eat, who you will be nice to, what outfit you will wear, and how hard you will work.

Our emotions rule us because we have rooted them in daily pressures, our circumstances, and other people's opinions instead of rooting them in a foundation of love from our Heavenly Father. When God called us to be in this world but not of it (John 15:19), that also included our emotions. God calls us to live beyond our emotions. We simply can't allow our emotions to dictate how we should live our lives. They're simply not reliable because they are based on what is in front of us at any given time. Our emotions are fleeting.

So does that mean we should not feel? Of course not. God wants our emotions to be grounded in Him. The next time you feel your emotions taking over, stop to pray and turn them over to God. Our emotional health is directly linked to our level of trust. Purpose to spend more time with Him and our feelings will be transformed into convictions and Godly wisdom about our health and all other areas of our lives.

Though our emotions may rage out of control, peace is a gift that can only be found when we seek the heart of God.

Action:

Pray that your emotions will be brought under God's submission.

Validation:

"Feeling trapped and feeling overwhelmed by needing to tie up so many loose ends each day."

"Stress, loneliness, anger, feeling sad, all of these emotions have led me to overeat, or just to continue eating when I was not hungry."

"Stress, anxiety, loneliness, and more! I probably eat for EVERY emotion I experience. However, it feels different for happy vs. sad emotions. For the sad ones, I just stuff and stuff and stuff, and it doesn't matter what I'm eating and it doesn't matter if I'm full. For the happy ones, I eat too much of food that I really like because it tastes so good to me!"

Meditation:

"In your anger do not sin... Do not let the sun go down while you are still angry, and do not give the devil a foothold."
(Ephesians 4:26–27 NIV)

When you make excuses you feed the devil

Inspiration:

"Feel your feelings, don't feed them."
~ Cathy Morenzie

Loren
DAgle
when you say!
(Saug)

Declaration:

Him who the Son sets free is free indeed! I rejoice because I am free from bondage. I am free from emotional eating. I am free to be me, created in Your image and destined for greatness. I have the capacity to effectively deal with every situation and circumstance that my mind, people, or the enemy will throw my way.

Supplication:

Thank You, Lord for giving me what I need to rise above every difficult situation and circumstance that comes my way. I pray that I would always fully trust in You moment by moment instead of giving in to my old ways of emotional eating. I claim victory over that bondage, through You, Lord Jesus. Thank You for the freedom that comes from living in You! In your Name I pray. Amen!

Reflection:

1. Meditate on the truth that God is your peace in the midst of your raging emotions. Allow Him to be your anchor when you're feeling emotional.

"To set the mind on the Spirit is life and peace."
(Romans 8:6)

"You keep him in perfect peace whose mind is stayed on you, because he trusts in you."
(Isaiah 26:3)

_____

_____

_____

_____

_____

_____

2. How do your emotions sabotage your health regimen? Ask the Holy Spirit to make you conscious of your emotions and then bring them under submission to God. *"We demolish arguments and every pretension that sets itself up against the knowledge of God, and we take captive every thought to make it obedient to Christ."* (2 Corinthians 10:2)

"Search me, God, and know my heart;
test me and know my anxious thoughts."
(Psalm 129:23)

_____

_____

_____

_____

_____

3. Seek the peace that comes from God. Refuse to be tossed to and fro at the whim of your emotions and stand firm in God's Word to keep you stable and peaceful. Instead of turning to food, make your requests to God.

"The Lord is at hand; do not be anxious about any-
thing, but in everything by prayer and supplication
with thanksgiving let your requests be made known
to God. And the peace of God, which surpasses all
understanding, will guard your hearts and your
minds in Christ Jesus."
(Philippians 4:5-7)

_____

_____

_____

_____

_____

Day 16:
2 hurs

PRAYER OF POSITIVE SELF-ESTEEM

Devotion:

Today, pray for the courage and confidence to be who God called you to be. Pray for self-esteem grounded in Christ.

One of the greatest testimonies we could ever give is to have the boldness and courage to live exactly how God called us to live. We would not try to puff ourselves up to be who we're not and we would not dumb ourselves down so we can hide in obscurity and never let our light shine. Sadly we move between these two extremes, looking for love and acceptance from a world standard that, no matter how hard we try, we will never measure up to anyway. So we turn to food to fill our needs and then turn to diets and weight loss gimmicks to help us stop turning to food and so the crazy cycle continues.

God is not concerned about what we look like on the outside, He's concerned with our hearts. God longs for us to love Him and be loved by Him. When we can understand this, our self-confidence will be through the roof! Our self-esteem comes from knowing that we are loved lavishly by God and He created us in His image. Let that be our main reason to hold ourselves in high esteem!

Action:

Pray for the courage and confidence to be who God called you to be.

Validation:

"I kind of copped out on answering this yesterday because I didn't want to even think about it. In many ways, the root issue is that I don't love myself. I tend to be overly critical and judgmental of me. I don't extend the same grace to myself that God extends to me, and I extend to others. I talk to myself, and about myself, in ways I would never talk to, or about, someone else. So, now I've taken a moment to look at me through the eyes of loving me because I am lovable. That right there is a key breakthrough that I must carry in my heart consistently. So, 10 things I love about myself: I love encouraging others, and myself, in the Word of God.

I love writing devotionals.

I love writing Scripture-based prayers and faith confessions.

I love giving and actively look for opportunities to bless others.

I love being six-feet tall!

I love having wash and go hair—no fuss, no muss.

I love that I am comfortable not wearing makeup.

I love having even skin tone.

I am a great friend, loyal, giving, and compassionate.

I am an excellent listener, practicing active listening—listening to hear and not listening to respond."

"I am loyal and trustworthy, loving, caring, pretty eyes, nice personality, good friend, good listener. As you can see I can't think of too many things good about myself, there's that low self-esteem. I know that because I am made in the likeness of Christ that I am beautiful."

"Great smile, loyal, loving, empathic, compassionate, fighter, passionate, funny, smart, encourager, and giver of great hugs."

Meditation:

"We even saw giants there, the descendants of Anak.
Next to them we felt like grasshoppers...!"
(Numbers 13:33 NLT)

Inspiration:

"Self-esteem is made up primarily of two things:
feeling lovable and feeling capable."
~ Jack Canfield

Declaration:

I am fearfully and wonderfully made. I am the apple of Your eye. There is no condemnation for those who are in Christ Jesus, because through Christ Jesus the Spirit set me free from the power of sin. I can certainly conquer this stronghold and any other one that will come my way, in Your matchless Name!

Supplication:

Dear Lord, I speak Your truth into my life. When You say that I am fearfully and wonderfully made I know You mean it! I release any bad thoughts of myself and only claim who I am in you. Help me to focus on my good qualities and leave it up to You to convict me of what needs to change. Your Word says that we are to love our neighbors as ourselves, so in order to be a more loving person I am going to start loving me and take care of myself. I do this as an offering to You. Amen!

Reflection:

1. Meditate on what the Bible teaches us about where to derive our confidence and self-esteem from.

> "For you formed my inward parts; you knitted me together in my mother's womb. I praise you, for I am fearfully and wonderfully made. Wonderful are your works; my soul knows it very well."
> (Psalm 139:13-14)

> "But the Lord said to Samuel, 'Do not look on his appearance or on the height of his stature, because I

have rejected him. For the Lord sees not as man sees:
man looks on the outward appearance,
but the Lord looks on the heart.'"
(1 Samuel 16:7)

_____

_____

_____

_____

_____

_____

_____

2. Ask God to show you what you look like in His eyes. What does He say about you? Ask Him what he thinks of you.

_____

_____

_____

_____

_____

_____

3. Reflect on the areas of your life where you're not taking action because you lack the self-esteem and confidence. Ask the Holy Spirit to empower you.

_____

_____

_____

_____

_____

_____

4. Fill in the blank: If I had more self-esteem I would... Ask the Holy Spirit to empower you to carry it out and then pray about the first step you will take to make it happen.

_____

_____

_____

_____

_____

_____

_____

Day 17:

PRAYER FOR SELF-CONTROL

Devotion:

Today, pray that God will empower you to control yourself.

Lack of self-control is one of the biggest frustrations we experience when we try to lose weight. How is it possible to feel so powerless over something so small as an ounce of chocolate? Or how is it that we can control ourselves 'perfectly' for 21 days straight and then completely lose control and go the opposite direction in the blink of an eye? It's because we need to refine our definition of self-control.

God's ways are radically different than the world's. The world tells us that we must have self-control and that we should look to our own strength as our source. But God flips this concept upside-down. He puts a higher value on those who acknowledge their inability to control themselves. When we acknowledge our weakness we gain the help of an Almighty, all-loving, ever-present God. Need to control your eating? Stop looking for willpower in yourself and look to God as your strength. In other words, the real secret to self-control is God-control.

Action:

Pray for God's control in your life instead of trying to control yourself in your own strength.

Validation:

"I feel the most vulnerable at work. I am a public school teacher and some days are very tough—unruly children, angry parents, and unreasonable expectations from administration. I have very little control over these things. I can only control my response to them and, unfortunately, it sometimes results in stress-eating."

"I struggle so much with getting enough sleep and rest. I've been trying to get to bed by 9:30–10:00. Last night I stayed up until around 12 doing nothing, just watching random clips on YouTube and Facebook. Lack of sleep hinders me from waking up refreshed in the mornings so I can exercise and do my daily devotional. Through this video today I saw how I'm sabotaging myself."

"I feel most vulnerable when I'm overwhelmed with my to-do list... I start to look around for a diversion and usually find myself in the kitchen. Another vulnerable time is after my husband has had an anger episode and I need comfort. I'm slowly learning to pray immediately in those moments instead."

Meditation:

"Be self-controlled and alert. Your enemy the devil
prowls around like a roaring lion looking for
someone to devour."
(1 Peter 5:8 NIV)

Inspiration:

"God has equipped you to handle difficult things.
In fact, He has already planted the seeds of discipline

and self-control inside you. You just have to water
those seeds with His Word to make them grow!"
~ Joyce Meyer

Declaration:

I stand firm against the enemy and he flees. I keep my eyes fixed on You, God, because You are the author and perfecter of my faith. I stand firm in Your Word. It is my sword and my shield. Your Word is a light unto my feet and a light unto my path. It brings me comfort, protection, and strength in times of need.

Supplication:

Dear Lord, please show me what causes me to lose my self-control in my life, especially with food. Lord, I want to operate in the purpose You have for me and not in a world of extremes. Thank You, Lord, for all that I am learning about making healthy lifestyle changes. Thank You for the changes I see happening in my life! In Your Name I pray. Amen!

Reflection:

1. Reflect on what the Bible says about self-control. What is God telling you? *"For it is we who are the circumcision, we who serve God by his Spirit, who boast in Christ Jesus, and who put no confidence in the flesh."* (Philippians 3:3)

"For whoever wants to save their life will lose it,
but whoever loses their life for me will find it."
(Matthew 16:25)

_____

_____

_____

_____

_____

_____

_____

2. How have you been trying to control your weight in your own strength? Why do you think you're doing it?

_____

_____

_____

_____

_____

_____

_____

3. Pray for the strength and courage to let go of your need to control, and allow yourself to find your strength in God.

"That is why, for Christ's sake, I delight in weaknesses,
in insults, in hardships, in persecutions, in difficulties.
For when I am weak, then I am strong."
(2 Corinthians 10:12)

_____

_____

_____

_____

_____

_____

_____

_____

_____

_____

_____

_____

Day 18:
Sat

THE PRAYER FOR FOCUS

Devotion:

Today, pray that you would keep your eyes fixed on the Lord and not on what you don't want.

There's a principle that states that what you focus on expands. Imagine if you were to apply this principle to your weight. Based on this theory, you would end up weighing more! Isn't that what happens to many of us? Despite all of the crazy diets and gimmicks, we often end up weighing more than we started. It's because we waste so much time focusing on what we don't want!

Here's a radical thought: what if you stopped focusing so much on your weight? What if you focused on being healthy and whole; on living out your life purpose; on being a light wherever you go? Focus on living a life that reflects your love for God and His love for you. Focus on what you want, not on what you don't want. When you choose to focus your life on Christ, He will do magnificent things in you today. Follow the path of focus Jesus laid out for you as you choose to be about our Father's business.

Action:

Pray that you would keep your eyes fixed on the Lord and not your problems.

Validation:

"I can spend too much time on Facebook, TV, and the phone. Setting a timer could help me focus better with my time. Sometimes I'll get in my car, take a short drive, and let good music relax me. It's such a great mood enhancer for me also."

"I lose focus when I am too busy and don't spend as much time with God as I need to. I can guard against this by praying about how I use my time and preserving enough time, first thing every morning, to listen to God and study His Word. Renewing my mind by praying and reading scriptures throughout the day will also help me stay focused."

"I lose focus when my routine is changed. I'm a creature of habit and find it difficult to continue with my health habits when things get disrupted. How can I guard against this? I suppose I'll need to just "go with the flow" and get back to routine as quickly as possible without deciding to just throw in the towel altogether."

Meditation:

"...Did you not know that I must be about
my Father's business?"
(Luke 2:49 NKJV)

Inspiration:

"When trouble comes, focus on God's ability
to care for you."
~ Charles Stanley

Declaration:

I have the mind of Christ. My mind is set on the spirit which is life and peace. My mind is being renewed day by day. The Holy Spirit lives in me and quickens me to do His will.

Supplication:

Dear Lord, Your grace is sufficient for me, Your power is made perfect in my weakness, and I give You the praise and glory! Lord, help me to stay focused on You so that the goal of a healthy weight will be attainable. May I keep my eyes always on You and not the difficult circumstances in my life. This way I won't sink back into my old ways and habits. In Your Holy Name I pray. Amen.

Reflection:

1. Spend some time and reflect on the life of Jesus. "...*knew you not that I must be about my Father's business?*" (Luke 2:49)

> "*Have this mind among yourselves, which is yours in Christ Jesus, who, though he was in the form of God, did not count equality with God a thing to be grasped, but emptied himself, by taking the form of a servant, being born in the likeness of men. And being found in human form, he humbled himself by becoming obe-dient to the point of death, even death on a cross.*"
> (Philippians 2:5–8)

_____

_____

_____

_____

_____

_____

_____

_____

2. What are all the ways you focus on your weight? Weighing on the scale? Critiquing yourself in the mirror? Starting a new diet? Ask the Holy Spirit to help you replace all of these habits with ones that will shift your focus to God.

_____

_____

_____

_____

_____

_____

_____

_____

3. Renew your mind today and receive a fresh anointing to center your life around Christ and not on your weight.

> *"For those who live according to the flesh set their*
> *minds on the things of the flesh, but those who live*
> *according to the Spirit set their minds on the things*
> *of the Spirit. For to set the mind on the flesh is death,*
> *but to set the mind on the Spirit is life and peace. For*
> *the mind that is set on the flesh is hostile to God, for*
> *it does not submit to God's law; indeed, it cannot.*
> *Those who are in the flesh cannot please God."*
> (Romans 8:5-8)

_____

_____

_____

_____

_____

_____

_____

_____

_____

_____

Day 19 :
Sun

PRAYER FOR STRATEGIC PARTNERSHIPS

Devotion:

Today pray for Godly friendships, accountability, and support in your health and weight- releasing journey.

Jesus summed up our purpose here on earth with these two statements: Love God and love people. Jesus teaches us that these two partnerships are crucial for our lives here on earth. They will be the cornerstone for your weight loss success as well as every other area of your life.

So often our pride will have us try to lose weight on our own. We simply cannot fathom the thought of people knowing that we're on yet another diet, or that we're still at this weight loss thing after so many failed attempts.

Accountability calls you to a higher standard when you don't feel like being your best. It increases your prayer power and gives you a safe space to be transparent and vulnerable, yet it does not let you off the hook when you're slipping. God has called us to be in relationship with Him and others, so don't overlook this treasure on your journey towards better health. But relationships do not happen in a vacuum—seek them out, pray for them as often as the Spirit leads, and continue to pray for their success as they pray for yours.

Action:

Pray for Godly friendships and accountability partners.

Validation:

"My husband has agreed to be my accountability partner. He will encourage me on my daily walk."

"My daughter—she doesn't slack or make excuses for doing exercise or eating nutritiously. I'm so grateful she's in my life!"

"My accountability partner is my good friend and neighbor. We talk almost every day and I've shared this journey so far with her. She is caring and giving and she gives me truth."

Meditation:

"He who walks with wise men will be wise, but the companion of fools will be destroyed."
(Proverbs 13:20 NKJV)

Inspiration:

"Accountability breeds response–ability."
~ Stephen Covey

Declaration:

I confess my sins to another as You have instructed. I thank You for my partners, and as iron sharpens iron we sharpen each other. We stand in agreement to manifest what You have already done in Heaven right here on earth! Your Word says where two or three are gathered, there You are in the midst, so we decree and declare that Your presence strengthens and empowers us.

Supplication:

Dear Lord, thank You for this opportunity to have an accountability partner. You know I need this support if I am going to succeed. May I in turn be support to them. Build us up in You, Lord. May we be transparent, and our focus be on You and Your will for our lives. Let us always speak the truth in love. In Your Name I pray. Amen!

Reflection:

1. Reflect on what the Bible says about accountability and partnerships. What is it teaching you?

> *"Walk with the wise and become wise, for a companion of fools suffers harm."*
> (Proverbs 13:20)

> *"As iron sharpens iron, so one person sharpens another."*
> (Proverbs 27:17)

_____

_____

_____

_____

_____

_____

_____

"For where two or three gather in my name,
there am I with them."
(Matt. 18:20)

2. God has created us to be in fellowship with our fellow sisters and brothers in Christ. How can you reach out to someone and support them on their health journey?

_____

_____

_____

_____

_____

_____

3. Accountability requires transparency and honesty. What are you afraid to tell someone in your life, out of fear that you will be judged in relation to your health journey? Pray for the strength to be transparent then share it with them as the Holy Spirit leads you.

_____

_____

_____

_____

_____

_____

_____

_____

_____

_____

_____

_____

_____

Day 20:
mon

PRAYER FOR PRIORITIZING

Devotion:

Today, pray that you would establish and maintain your priorities as you put boundaries around your time.

How would you rank your life? Most of us would not hesitate to say God is first, but then what would you put second? Your husband, children, career, ministry? What if I told you that you should come first? For many of us Christian women the idea of putting yourself first may sound selfish and contrary to what we've been taught, but think about it. How can you take care of anyone else if you don't have the physical, spiritual, mental, and emotional health and strength for yourself? Here's the right priority: Spend time with God and get filled with His love, then you will have lots of love to give away. Otherwise, you can't give away what you don't have.

Once you put yourself as a priority, pray and ask God to show you how to put boundaries around your time so that you can keep the main things the main things. Pray against distraction and pay attention to what sucks up your time. The more mindful you become about how you spend your time, the better you will become at focusing on what's important.

Action:

Pray that you will establish boundaries around your time and learn to prioritize God and yourself.

Validation:

"Much as I love my husband, daughter and friends, I need time alone to recharge and be the best I can be. I need to schedule in that time of quiet reflection even if I have to get in my car and flee the people I love to get it! I can manage all the rest of my life better if I have regular time on my own."

"I am going to say no to sleeping late and say no to excessive time on the internet and watching TV. I will say yes to consistently exercising 3-4 times a week, consistently reading my Bible every day, and I will say yes to increasing my daily intake of water."

"Saying no to others when they are imposing on my time. I give so much of myself and I always leave myself out by attending to their every need. It is time for me to focus on myself."

Meditation:

"You expected much, but see, it turned out to be little...Because of my house, which remains a ruin, while each of you is busy with his own house."
(Haggai 1:9 NIV)

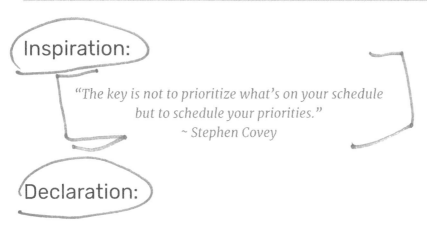

Inspiration:

*"The key is not to prioritize what's on your schedule
but to schedule your priorities."*
~ Stephen Covey

Declaration:

Father, we thank You that when we put You first You teach us how to prioritize. My steps are ordered by You. I seek Your Kingdom above all else, and in doing so You teach me how to make the most of my day. In all I do, I worship You. My time is in Your hands and You have blessed it and given me good success.

Supplication:

Dear Lord, thank You for using all my decisions, even the poor ones. Lord, I want to be on the right course, so I'm going to read Your scriptures and reach out to you each day. Lord, I want my plans for my life to be Your plans. Guide me in all I do. I pray that others would see You in me as I seek to do Your will. I want to take action steps in the right direction, and succeed in becoming a healthy person. I ask for Your richest blessings on my life and everyone I know! Amen.

Reflection:

1. Reflect on the importance of loving yourself well so you can love others. How well could you love your neighbor if you don't have any love for yourself?

"You shall love your neighbor as yourself."
(Mark 12:31)

_____

_____

_____

_____

_____

_____

_____

_____

2. We often get so caught up doing other things that we can easily put ourselves at the bottom of the priority list. How is God calling you to make yourself a priority?

_____

_____

_____

_____

_____

_____

3. Take a moment and surrender your priority list to God. Ask Him to order your steps so that you can keep Him first, you second, and others after.

_____

_____

_____

_____

_____

_____

_____

_____

_____

_____

_____

_____

_____

_____

Day 21:

PRAYER FOR PERSEVERANCE

Devotion:

Today, pray for perseverance on this journey. Pray that you will not grow weary and that you will continue in the Lord's strength.

Most of us can muster up the strength to do something difficult or sacrificial for a period of time—we've all done it. We can do a challenge for 21 days, or go to the gym consistently for the first weeks in January, but what happens when the willpower runs out, as it always does? What happens when we're no longer feeling motivated and inspired? That's when we need God's power to help us persevere.

Too often we see change as a one-time deal. We identify the problem, we try to fix it, we realize it's not as easy as we thought, we experience setbacks, and we give up and say it didn't work. But that's not how the heart of God operates. God is continually transforming us day by day. There is never a point when we're done. Sure, we may achieve our ideal weight, but God wants so much more from us than to achieve a certain weight on the scale. Everything that we do has eternal implications, and that's why we will always keep on learning, growing, and drawing closer to God.

As you wrap up this challenge, continue to maintain your daily conversations with God. Make prayer an ongoing conversation with God for your health, as well as all other areas of your life.

Action:

Pray that you will not grow weary on the journey—that you will continue in the Lord's strength.

- Spending time with Him

- Prayer Procrastination

- Excuse-making

- Blaming

- Self-Esteem

- Staying Focused

- Slowing Down

- Getting to the root of your weight loss challenges

- Accountability

- Exercising

- Changing your diet

- Other

Meditation:

"Blessed is the man who remains steadfast under trial, for when he has stood the test he will receive the crown of life, which God has promised to those who love him."
(James 1:12 ESV)

Inspiration:

"Failure plus failure plus failure equals success. You only fail when you quit."
~ Jack Hyles

Declaration:

We decree that we will remain steadfast in our assignment to strengthen our temples. We declare that we will not quit, not give up, not let up, and not hold back. We look to You for strengthening in times of testing and trial, and stand on Your Word. When we are weak, then we are truly strong in You.

Supplication:

I wish I had this

Dear Lord, thank You for this opportunity to have an accountability partner. You know I need this support if I am going to succeed. May I in turn be support to them. Build us up in You, Lord. May we be transparent, and our focus be on You and Your will for our lives. Let us always speak the truth in love. In Your Name I pray. Amen!

Reflection:

1. Spend some time reflecting on how God wants to continually work in your life to transform you and your weight loss. *"And we all, who with unveiled faces contemplate the Lord's glory, are being transformed into his image with ever-increasing glory, which comes from the Lord, who is the Spirit."* (2 Corinthians 3:18)

> *"Fear not, for I am with you; be not dismayed, for I am your God; I will strengthen you, I will help you, I will uphold you with my righteous right hand."*
> (Isaiah 41:10)

_____

_____

_____

_____

_____

_____

_____

_____

2. Ask the Holy Spirit to give you the discipline and strength to continually seek after the things of God, and to continue seeking God's heart. Ask Him to show you what's next in your journey towards better heath and wholeness.

"You will seek me and find me when you seek me
with all your heart."
(Jeremiah 29:13)

_____

_____

_____

_____

_____

_____

3. Reflect upon the process of change. It's never in a straight line as we would like it to be. Make the commitment today to stay the course by continually seeking after God's heart and purpose in your heart that you will walk with God on this journey always.

Whether you turn to the right or to the left, your ears will hear a voice behind you, saying, 'This is the way; walk in it.'"

_____

_____

_____

_____

_____

_____

THANK YOU

Thank you for being motivated, courageous, inquisitive and committed to go deeper in your health journey and uncover the missing piece- Christ! I pray that these principles have been as much of a blessing to you as they have been for me and the hundreds of thousands of women around the world that have experienced what it means to include God in their health and weight-releasing journey.

If you've been blessed by this book, then please don't keep it a secret!

There are millions of women who need to hear this message. Please take a moment to leave an honest book review so more people can discover this book as well.

This book has laid out a great foundation for you, but there's so much more for you to discover. Please keep in touch with me so that you can stay in this conversation and continue to make your health a priority--God's Way. I'll send you a free copy of my '3 Steps to Overcoming Emotional Eating' guide, and a discount for an online version of this devotion, when you enroll for my weekly emails on successful weight loss, God's way.

praypowerfullyloseweightbonus.com

Appendix

Photocopy or cut out the declaration(s) you want
to recite and place in a prominent place you'll
see them daily. You can also print out a .pdf of
these declarations from:

www.cathymorenzie.com/declarations

Declarations

•Day 1: For the Journey

I walk in wisdom to set realistic goals that glorify You. I submit my goals and plans to You and I trust You to show me the way. My goals align with my Heavenly Father's, and are bathed in the Word of God. I declare that my goals will come to fruition. As I draw close to You I am successful and victorious, in the Name of Jesus.

• Day 2: For Your Willingness

I am as bold as a lion. I can endure to the end because You are my strength and shield. I have the capacity for victorious living. I operate in excellence and purpose to complete every task that I set out to do. I can do all things through Christ who gives me strength. There is no temptation that can overtake me because You give me the strength to bear up under it. My sacrifice is my form of worship to You, so I do it with peace and gratitude.

Day 3: For Your Actions

All things work together for good. My pain will turn into laughter, my cross will be exchanged for a crown, and my mourning will be turned into dancing. I am blessed and I am a blessing. My disappointments of the past will be turned into testimonies, in the Name of Jesus.

Day 4 - For Understanding the Process

Thank you for your promises. I am making progress. From victory to victory, success to success, I am getting stronger each day. I am more than an overcomer. I am unstoppable, and I am advancing in everything I put my mind to.

Day 5 - For Submitting to God

I walk in Your presence today and I choose to honor You, God, by what I eat and in all I do. I submit my weight, my health, and my body to You. I walk with courage, discipline, and perseverance in times of testing and temptation. I am blessed and prosperous in You.

Day 6 - For Your Prayer Life

I thank You that I don't have to be worried or anxious about anything. I bring my request to You with thanksgiving and stand in confidence that You will bring it to fruition. I submit my request to You, who are able to do exceeding abundantly above all that I can ask or think.

Day 7 - For the Power to Choose

I am dead to sin. Your strength and grace have changed me and renewed me. I have a new life in You and do things that lead to holiness and joy. The power of your life-giving Spirit has freed me from the power of sin. Your Spirit that controls my mind has given me life and peace.

Day 8 - For the Power to Think Positively

I have the faith to move mountains. The Holy Spirit in me has made the impossible possible. I am more than a conqueror, and I can overcome any obstacle that stands in my path. No weapon formed against me shall prosper. I am constantly making progress. I am a success.

Day 9 - For the Power to Raise Your Awareness

I love You, Lord, and thank You for Your Spirit which lives in me. My mind is set on things above. I become more and more like You each day. I am created in Your image. I make responsible choices and decisions. I have the ability to solve my problems with You as my guide. I take authority over this day, in the Name of Jesus.

Day 10 - For the Power of Insight

Have mercy on me, Christ. You have searched me, God, and helped me uncover my anxious thoughts. I now begin the process of rooting them out forever. I thank You for replacing my old behaviors with new ones that are pleasing in Your eyes. Because of Your love I am dead to sin. I boldly take hold of Your power which gives me victory over sin.

Day 11 - For the Power to Overcome Limiting Beliefs

Your promises are for eternity. Every generational curse and everything spoken against my health is broken in the Name of Jesus. I declare that I am in sound health in my body, mind, and spirit. I am strong and courageous, and successful in everything I do. I meditate on Your Word day and night. Him who the Son sets free is free indeed, and I declare my freedom in You.

Day 12 - For the Power to Overcome Excuse Making

Father, You've clothed me with strength and honor; You've empowered me to be strong and courageous. I reclaim my power in You by taking 100% responsibility for my thoughts and actions. I am blessed with the Holy Ghost to accomplish my weight loss goals. I will have a testimony, in the Name of Jesus.

Day 13 - For the Power to Overcome Blaming

Father, forgive me for usurping my responsibility to You for my weight loss and wellness. Excellent health is mine, energy and vitality are mine. I am designed to reach higher levels of health from victory to victory, glory to glory, in the Name of Jesus!

Day 14 - For the Power to Overcome Procrastination

I seek Your Kingdom above all else. I put You before my agendas, my timelines, and my priorities. I walk in faith and not fear. I walk in power, victory, and a sound mind. I do everything on time and in order. All my steps are ordered by You.

Day 15 - For the Power to Overcome Emotional Eating

Him who the Son sets free is free indeed! I rejoice because I am free from bondage. I am free from emotional eating. I am free to be me, created in Your image and destined for greatness. I have the capacity to effectively deal with every situation and circumstance that my mind, people, or the enemy will throw my way.

Day 16 - For the Power to Overcome Poor Self-Image

I am fearfully and wonderfully made. I am the apple of Your eye. There is no condemnation for those who are in Christ Jesus, because through Christ Jesus the Spirit set me free from the power of sin. I can certainly conquer this stronghold, and any other one that will come my way, in Your matchless Name!

Day 17 - For the Power of Self-Control

I stand firm against the enemy and he flees. I keep my eyes fixed on You, God, because You are the author and perfecter of my faith. I stand firm in Your Word. It is my sword and my shield. Your Word is a light unto my feet and a light unto my path. It brings me comfort, protection, and strength in times of need.

Day 18 - For the Power to Stay Focused

I have the mind of Christ. My mind is set on the Spirit, which is life and peace. My mind is being renewed day by day. The Holy Spirit lives in me, and quickens me to do His will.

Day 19 - For Strategic Partnerships

I confess my sins to another as You have instructed. I thank You for my partners, and as iron sharpens iron we sharpen each other. We stand in agreement to manifest what You have already done in Heaven right here on earth! Your Word says where two or three are gathered there You are in the midst, so we decree and declare that Your presence strengthens and empowers us.

Day 20 - For the Power to Prioritize

Father, I thank You that when I put You first You teach me how to prioritize. My steps are ordered by You. I seek Your Kingdom above all else, and in doing so You teach me how to make the most of my day. In all I do, I worship You. My time is in Your hands, and You have blessed it and given me good success.

Day 21 - For the Power to Overcome— Staying the Course

I decree that I will remain steadfast in my assignment to strengthen my temple. I declare that I will not quit, not give up, not let up, and not hold back. I look to You for strengthening in times of testing and trial, and stand on Your Word. When I am weak, then I am truly strong in You.

Not sure how to pray?
Use these prayers as a guideline or inspiration as
you develop confidence in your own prayer life.

Prayers

Day 1 - Prayer for the Journey

Dear Lord, I want to glorify You in my body because it is Your temple. I submit myself and my goals to You. I know when I am in alignment with Your will and purpose for my life, I will be successful! Lord, give me the courage to take steps every day towards fulfilling my health goals and becoming the person You created me to be. In Your glorious Name I pray. Amen!

Day 2 - Prayer for Sacrificial Living

Lord, You have given me the power and strength to develop a healthier lifestyle that glorifies You. Teach me how to give up my own unhealthy desires in order to glorify You and my body. I can endure the temptations because You are my strength and my shield. I can spend time planning to eat healthfully and exercise because You have given me the capacity for victorious living. I find complete healing in You! Thank You, Lord, for blessing me in every way! In Jesus' Name. Amen.

Day 3 - Prayer for Action

Dear Lord, I pray that I would not sit idly by in the comfort of overeating and not exercising. You've shown me that the price is too high to pay. Lord, You have given me a vision for what my life will be like when I am totally surrendered to You and I am at a healthy weight, and the costs involved if I don't.

I choose a better way. Strengthen my mind and will, Lord. In Your Name I pray. Amen.

✓ Day 4 - Prayer for Progress

Dear Lord, some days the progress feels so slow and seems like it will take forever to reach a healthy weight. Thank You for reminding me that the process and its lessons are just as important as the goal. I am getting stronger and stronger each day. I am learning new things about You and myself each day, and I am more than an overcomer. I have victory in You, Lord! Thank You for your love, grace, and blessings. In Jesus' Name. Amen

✓ Day 5 - Prayer for Submission

Dear Lord, I come to You humbly and admit to You that I can't release this unhealthy weight on my own. I've tried for so long and in so many different ways. Lord, I open my heart and mind to Your prompting as I submit to You. I invite You to lead me in this process. I commit to doing Your will. In Your Name I pray. Amen.

✓ Day 6 - Prayer for God's Presence

Dear Lord, it is such a comfort to know that You are always right there! All I need to do is just start talking to You and You listen with such love and compassion. I need You, Lord, now more than ever. These patterns of unhealthy eating and not exercising are so ingrained in me. I need Your healing touch in my life and I need Your guidance. Lord, I want to be a blessing to You and glorify You in my body. Thank You that I don't need to fret over how this will transpire, because You have this all under control and I submit myself to You. In Jesus' Name. Amen.

Day 7 - Prayer for Making Right Choices

Dear Lord, thank You that I am a new creation in You. I pray that my mind and heart would grasp this and that I would rest in Your amazing transforming power and love. Lord, please reveal to me what small step You would have me take to make a healthy change in my life. I get so overwhelmed when I try to do it in my own strength, so I'm giving this all to You. I also turn discouragement and fear over to You right now and claim the power I have in You. I can do all things through You because You give me strength! In Jesus' Name. Amen.

Day 8 - Prayer for Speaking Life Over Yourself

Dear Lord, I am strong and courageous because of You. I am fearfully and wonderfully made! So Lord, I am boldly asking in faith to be an overcomer in the areas I struggle with in my life, especially with food, exercise, and negative self-talk. I pray that You would help me to see myself as You see me. Although my faith is as small as a mustard seed, You say in Your Word that this is enough to move a mountain! In You and through You, I am making progress. May I bring You glory as people see the changes in my life. Thank You for coming alongside me and being my rock! I ask these things in the powerful Name of Jesus. Amen.

Day 9 - Prayer for Conscious Living

Dear Lord, I choose to live consciously in the here and now. I will check in with You hour by hour and trust that You will show me how to be more aware of my eating patterns. I am being transformed and renewed day by day by living my life in You, and by keeping my mindset on things above. I pray, Lord, for continued strength to make wise decisions regarding my health. I know I can do all things through You. And by Your grace, I am becoming more and more like You every day. In your Name I pray. Amen.

Day 10 - Prayer for Insight

Dear Lord, I do what I don't want to do, and don't do what I want to do, but that is because I am trying to do this in my own power. Lord, I submit my recurring patterns to You. I submit my whole life to You. Your ways are so much better than mine. Help me come to grips with my sinful nature so that I may abide in You fully. Replace my fears and faults with Christ's freedom. You are the only one who can give true lasting victory from the bondage of unhealthy eating and lack of exercise. I want to glorify You, Lord, with my life! In Your Name, Amen.

Day 11 - Prayer to Overcome Limiting Beliefs

Dear Lord, I pray that in Your mighty power You would break every generational curse and everything spoken against my health. Lord, You want healing and wholeness in my life but I can't do this in my own strength. So, I lay my life and its brokenness at the foot of your cross. I declare victory in You. I am strong and courageous and successful in all that I do because You promise that those who the Son sets free are free indeed! In Your Name I pray. Amen!

• Day 12 - Prayer for Overcoming Excuses

Dear Lord, I have made excuses long enough. Yes, Lord, I want to get well! Show me what excuses are holding me back from glorifying You in my body, even ones I hold on to sub-consciously. You have empowered me with Your Holy Spirit, and I claim that power! I will take 100% responsibility for my thoughts and actions so that I will accomplish my goal of get-ting to a healthy weight. In Your Name I pray. Amen.

Day 13 - Prayer for Overcoming Blaming

Dear Lord, forgive me for playing the blame game. Thank You for revealing to me who and what I blame for my excess weight. I claim 100% responsibility right now! Forgive me for holding on to past hurts and faulty ideas. Lord, help me to for-give those I need to forgive and to let go of those past hurts and feelings that I have been holding on to for so long. Bring healing to those wounded areas of my heart. I claim excellent health and energy right now! In Your precious Name I pray. Amen.

Day 14 - Prayer for Overcoming Procrastination

Dear Lord, I want more of You and less of me. I put my pri-orities and time, and anything that I put before You, aside. Lord, You know my fears and all that hinders me from totally sur-rendering to You. Reveal to me those things that I'm not even aware of, and convict me of my procrastinating. I don't want anything holding me back from moving forward in victory towards my goal of a healthy weight and healthy body, so I claim victory in Your Holy Name! You give me power and a sound mind in order to be an overcomer. In Your Name I pray. Amen.

Day 15 - Prayer for Overcoming Emotional Eating

Thank You, Lord, for giving me what I need to rise above every difficult situation and circumstance that comes my way. I pray that I would always fully trust in You, moment by moment, instead of giving in to my old ways of emotional eating. I claim victory over that bondage through You, Lord Jesus. Thank You for the freedom that comes from living in You! In Your Name I pray. Amen.

Day 16 - Prayer for Self-Esteem

Dear Lord, I speak Your truth into my life. When You say that I am fearfully and wonderfully made I know You mean it! I release any bad thoughts of myself and only claim who I am in You. Help me to focus on my good qualities and leave it up to You to convict me of what needs to change. Your Word says that we are to love our neighbors as ourselves, so in order to be a more loving person I am going to start loving me and taking care of myself. I do this as an offering to You. In Jesus' Name. Amen.

Day 17 - Prayer for Self-Control

Dear Lord, please show me what causes me to lose my self-control in my life—especially with food. Lord, I want to operate in the purpose You have for me and not in a world of extremes. Thank You, Lord, for all that I am learning about making healthy lifestyle changes. Thank You for the changes I see happening in my life! In Your Name I pray. Amen.

Day 18 - Prayer for Focus

Dear Lord, Your grace is sufficient for me and Your power is made perfect in my weakness. I give You praise and glory! Lord, help me to stay focused on You so that the goal of a healthy weight will be attainable. May I keep my eyes always on You and not the difficult circumstances in my life; this way I won't sink back into my old ways and habits. In Your Holy Name I pray. Amen.

Day 19 - Prayer for Strategic Partnerships

Lord, we thank You that as we love and build one another up we ourselves are healed. Continue to teach us humility as we bear one another's burdens. Help us to be transparent before You and our fellow sisters so we can truly encounter the full-ness of the abundant life Jesus' death gives us. Build us up when no one else can, love us when we feel unloved, and fill us when we feel empty. As You fill our tanks, we will pay it forward and help our fellow sisters. In Your Name I pray. Amen.

Day 20 - Prayer for Prioritizing

Dear Lord, thank You for using all my decisions, even the poor ones. I want to be on the right course, so I'm going to read Your Scripture and reach out to You each day. Lord, I want my plans for my life to be Your plans. Guide me in all I do. I pray that others would see You in me as I seek to do Your will. I want to take action steps in the right direction and succeed in becoming a healthy person. I ask for Your richest blessings on my life and everyone I know! In the Name of your precious Son, Amen.

Day 21 - Prayer for Perseverance

Dear Lord, some days the progress feels so slow and seems like it will take forever to reach a healthy weight. Thank You for reminding me that the process and its lessons are just as important as the goal. I am getting stronger and stronger each day. I am learning new things about You and myself each day, and I am more than an overcomer. I have victory in You, Lord! Thank You for Your love, grace, and blessings. In Jesus' Name, Amen.

Other Healthy by Design Offerings

Healthy by Design (healthybydesignprogram.com) equips women to rely on God as their strength so they can live in freedom, joy, and peace. At the end of the day, that's what we really want. Let's be honest, if you never achieved that mythical, illusive number on the scale, but were fully able to live a life of freedom, joy, and peace, would that be enough? I know for me the answer is a resounding 'YES!!!'

We provide a multidimensional approach to releasing weight. It encompasses the whole person—spiritual, psychological, mental, nutritional, physical, and even hormonal! We believe that you must address the whole person—body, soul, and spirit. If you're looking for a program that just tells you what to eat and what exercises to do, this ain't it.

This program has helped thousands of women break free from all the roadblocks that have been hindering their weight loss success while discovering their identity in Christ.

Healthy by Design offers a variety of free and paid courses and programs. They include the following:

A YouVersion Bible Study

A free basic introduction to Step 1 of the WLGW program. To learn more, go to:

https://my.bible.com/reading-plans/4593-weight-loss-gods-way.com

Or from the YouVersion Bible App, click the bottom center, 'check-mark' button to open devotions, and search for 'Weight Loss God's Way or our other free devotionals:

Rest, Restore, and Rejuvenate

Praying for Your Health

The Weight Loss, God's Way Newsletter

Join the free *Weight Loss, God's Way* community and receive weekly posts designed to help you align your weight loss with God's Word. You'll also receive our Love Letters from God free download. To join the newsletter, sign up at:

lovegodloseweightbonus.com

The Membership Program

A done-for-you, step-by-step guide to the entire program. Dozens of bonus tools like group coaching calls, forums, and accountability groups. To become a *Weight Loss, God's Way* member, go to:

christianweightlossgodsway.com

Bible Studies for Churches and Small Groups

The membership program can also be experienced a la carte with a group of your friends or with your church. Take one of our three—to-six-week studies on a variety of health and weight-releasing topics. To learn more about starting a Bible study in your home or church, go to:

https://www.cathymorenzie.com/start-a-wlgw-group/

Books and Devotionals

You can find all of our *Healthy by Design* series of weight loss books here:

Christianweightlossbooks.com

Keynote Speaking

Want me to visit your hometown? Need a speaker for your annual conference or special event? My fun and practical approach to *Weight Loss, God's Way* will give your group clarity and focus to move toward their weight loss goals. To learn more or to book a speaking engagement, visit:

https://www.cathymorenzie.com/speaking/

Private Coaching

Prefer a more one-on-one approach? I have a few dedicated time slots available to coach you individually to help you fast-track your results. To learn more, go to:

https://www.cathymorenzie.com/coach-with-cathy-2/

Other Healthy by Design books by Cathy Morenzie:

Weight Loss, God's Way

21-Day Meal Plan

Love God, Lose Weight

Coming soon:

Breakthrough

Strong Faith, Strong Finish

Online programs by Cathy Morenzie:

Weight Loss, God's Way 21-Day Challenge:
21daysgodsway.com

5 Steps to Christian Weight Loss Course:
5stepscourse.com

Weight Loss, God's Way Membership:
christianweightlossgodsway.com

Pray Powerfully, Lose Weight
praypowerfullyloseweight.com

Love God, Lose Weight
lovegodloseweight.com

Strong Faith, Strong Finish
strongfaithstrongfinish.com

About The Author

Cathy is a noted personal trainer, author, blogger and presenter, and has been a leader in the faith/fitness industry for over a decade. Her impact has influenced thousands of people over the years to help them lose weight and develop positive attitudes about their bodies and fitness. Over the years, she has seen some of the most powerful and faith-filled people struggle with their health and their weight.

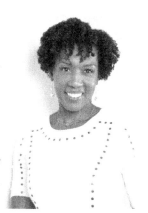

Cathy Morenzie herself—a rational, disciplined, faith-filled personal trainer—struggled with her own weight, emotional eating, self-doubt, and low self-esteem. She tried to change just about everything about herself for much of her life, so she knows what it's like to feel stuck. Every insecurity, challenge, and negative emotion that she experienced has equipped her to help other people who face the same struggles—especially women.

With her Healthy by Design books and Weight Loss, God's Way programs, Cathy has helped thousands to learn to let go of their mental, emotional, and spiritual bonds that have kept them stuck, and instead rely on their Heavenly Father for true release from their fears, doubts, stress, and anxiety. She also teaches people how to eat a sustainable, nutritious diet, and find the motivation to exercise.

Learn more at www.cathymorenzie.com.

Follow Cathy at:
https://www.facebook.com/weightlossgodsway/
https://www.youtube.com/user/activeimage1

Made in United States
Orlando, FL
02 April 2022

16421814R00096